Illegally Thin

By

RANDOM KNIGHT

Dedication

This book is dedicated to all those who suffer from excess weight or related problems and to all those dedicated to fighting the tyranny of agencies like the FDA.

A lie can travel halfway around the world while the truth is putting on its shoes. ~Mark Twain

Illegally Thin

By

RANDOM KNIGHT

The information provided in this publication should not be used to diagnose or treat any health problem, disease or condition. The writer and printers of this book make no medical claims for any products mentioned. This information is provided solely as a discussion of the substances listed, and the writers and printers/publishers of this book assume no responsibility for the use or misuse of any substances listed.

Always consult a qualified health care provider before beginning any weight loss or dietary change program. The statements contained herein have not been evaluated by the Food and Drug Administration and are not intended to diagnose, treat, cure or prevent any disease. The statements are for informational purposes only and are not meant to replace the services or recommendations of a physician or qualified health care practitioner.

You assume full responsibility for all of the health information contained within this publication. We cannot be held liable in any way for results stemming from the practical use of this information. Under no circumstances shall the writer/publisher/printer of this publication or the employees of the writer/printer/publisher or those of its affiliated organizations or any related individuals or entities be liable for damages of any kind arising from the use of this information, including, but not limited to, direct, indirect, special, consequential or punitive damages or lost profits.

This information is published under the First Amendment right to free speech and are intended as a discussion only. The writer/publisher/printers of this book are in no way encouraging the illegal use of any substances and do not suggest that anyone break any current laws. All information contained in this publication is for informational and educational purposes only and in no way substitutes for the advice of a qualified medical professional.

You expressly understand and agree that the author of this book shall not be liable to you for any direct, indirect, incidental, special, consequential or exemplary damages, including intangible losses, resulting from: the use or the inability to use any substances listed within, or any services or products of any third party; or statements or conduct of any third party.

Information and advice is based on the authors own experiences and research. Please get advice from your physician or other qualified health professional before taking supplements of any kind. The information provided in this publication is believed to be accurate based on the best judgment of the author.

ISBN: 978-0-615-26289-5

First Edition: February 2009

TABLE OF CONTENTS

A Friendly Warning from the Author

Be careful to read this book completely before researching this subject independently. There is a considerable amount of misinformation and hype about this chemical, and much of it is both negative and inaccurate. If you do not read this book before you do your own research, there is virtually a 100% chance that you will walk away confused and disillusioned. Consequently, it is a virtual certainty that you will never be able to take advantage of this chemical, or to promote its rightful return to use as a prescription medicine. To my knowledge, there is no other single source or document on this substance that, provides an objective critical analysis, that is carefully supported by clinical studies.

Other than the clinical studies and reports, mostly done decades ago, there is nowhere that you can find the objective truth about this substance. The assertions in this book are in substantial agreement with the conclusions regarding this chemical's safety and effectiveness of most, if not all of the clinical studies, I have researched.

This book promotes nothing but liberty and opportunity through knowledge of the truth. Read, learn, enjoy, and then decide for yourself.

FOREWORD

As I am writing this, I cannot help but notice the connection between my book's revelations and the calamites presently engulfing the American economy. Everyday there is news about the meltdown of the American financial system. Just last night, experts were saying that the single biggest problem contributing to our country's financial woes is that the national debt is really over 50 trillion dollars, not the 10 trillion or so that is reported on the news. These experts reported that both of these amounts are the Federal Government's own figures. The discrepancy is in what parts of the debt that both figures include. For instance, social security is not included in the bookkeeping totals for certain federal budget reports every year.

> "I don't think it is nearly as devastating in terms of human suffering as the corruption this book reveals"

Whichever number you believe, one thing is obvious: our government and our financial system have become corrupt. This is not at all surprising, considering that the power of a government office is an attractive target for those who seek control and money, without regard for the standards of right and wrong.

Governmental concentrations of power have always been used and abused to gain financial advantage for a few, at the expense of everyone else. The cumulative acts of governmental corruption, both by those in the government being corrupted and those doing the corrupting in the private sector have brought about the collapse of many of our nation's largest financial institutions. The ramifications of this greed and selfishness will play out in suffering and hardship for hundreds of millions of people for years to come. As bad as all of this fallout is

3

going to be from this present abuse of our financial system, I don't think it is nearly as devastating in terms of human suffering, as the corruption this book reveals.

The greed driven corruption that this book reveals does imply a huge cumulative financial cost to our nation, but the cost in human suffering, apart from economic ramifications, is even crueler. Let's cut to the chase; in the United States we have the technology, in the form of a certain chemical, to eradicate obesity and any kind of excess body fat. We have had this medical technology for decades. The federal government, specifically the FDA (Food and Drug Administration), is standing between the people of this country and this solution to obesity and other weight related problems.

This book is intended to remedy the current situation by making the American people aware of this substance they once had, but subsequently lost when the FDA banned it. If this chemical is returned to its status as a legal prescription drug, obesity and less serious weight problems could almost completely disappear. Please be patient, this book will prove everything I just stated and more.

For a moment just imagine what eradicating the scourge of excess body fat would mean. Obesity is the single biggest health crisis in America. Heart attack and stroke are the number one and three killers. Both are largely a consequence of obesity. Studies have also proven that being overweight can greatly increase the risk of multiple types of cancer. The health problems that obesity causes are almost endless.

> "Obesity is the single biggest health crisis in America"

If virtually all Americans who needed to were able to lose all of their excess body fat, how many health problems would diminish or disappear with that extra weight? No one can know for sure, but I would estimate between one third and one half of all health problems could be cured or alleviated.

There are other benefits as well. How much mental and emotional suffering would be alleviated? How much physical pain? How much inconvenience?

It would be a dream-come-true for millions upon millions of people. Imagine walking through a mall and every person you see is thin. The hundreds of millions of people suffering from the conditions that accompany excess body fat would have a tremendous load of difficulty and suffering lifted. While this dream is not a reality at the moment, it could be if the truth revealed in this book could motivate enough people to resist the stranglehold of special interests on the FDA, sufficiently to reverse its bad decision to ban this chemical.

I am absolutely convinced that this is one of the most, if not *the most* valuable chemical therapeutic discoveries ever. Aside from the many clinical studies and great deal of other information I encountered in my research, there is another reason I am convinced of this chemical's effectiveness and safety; I have used it myself. I lost an average of a little more than half a pound of fat a day (or over three pounds a week) with no negative side effects. I didn't have a lot of fat to spare either. I was six feet tall 181 pounds when I started. I dropped to 175 pounds and less than 10 percent body-fat in nine days of therapy with this chemical. I am at the same weight today.

> "I am absolutely convinced that this is one of the most, if not *the most* valuable chemical therapeutic discoveries ever"

I felt confident taking this substance because I knew it was safe and effective, based on the experience of clinicians, doctors, patients and hundreds of thousands of Americans who used it when it was legal. Additionally, my research on modern day underground use gave me an understanding of what to expect and proper precautions and protocols for using this therapy. I did not need to lose weight, but I wanted to have first-hand experience with this substance, before publishing this book. From a safety standpoint, I can tell you that I

5

would confidently recommend using this chemical for fat loss to my own children if they needed it. The only reservation I would have with recommending this substance is with advising anyone to break the laws regarding its use in the USA. I would recommend leaving the country or pursuing some other legal option so that anyone using DNP would not be breaking the current laws.

This book is divided into three parts. The first part explains this drug and the second provides clinical studies that back a variety of facts related to its usage, safety and benefits. I will also prove through common sense and documentation that everything I have told you is true.

Another way to describe the first part is that it is the revelation and advocacy of the assertion that the American people are being unjustly deprived of one of the most valuable and needed medical therapies ever discovered, because of special interest's greed and government corruption. I consider this first part of the book to be the most valuable and important part.

The chapter in the first half of the book that I consider the most interesting and informative is the "Arguments and Answers" chapter. If you like sarcasm, you might also find it to be the most entertaining. The chapter on my own usage is also of particular interest, because it begins by describing my own intellectual evolution on the benefits and risks of this chemical.

The second part consists of clinical reports and other types of technical and scientific data. The 1934 Stanford University report is the definitive work by the greatest experts on the subject.

The third part of this book is completely different. It deals with what I have learned from my research of modern underground use of this chemical. It is not an advocacy of anything. It is a report of my research. Nothing in that section should be seen as anything but a factual report of this underground use. It covers use protocols, dosage protocols, dose related side effects, first person usage logs relating peoples experience and results as well as other information regarding present day use of this substance for weight loss.

PART ONE

Background and Common Sense
The True Story of the Greatest Fat Reduction Substance Known to Man

The marvel of all history is the patience with which
men and women submit to burdens unnecessarily laid
upon them by their governments.
~William H. Borah

CHAPTER ONE

Description and History

The Basic Premise of this Book

What would you think, if I told you that there is a chemical that you can take to burn fifteen pounds of fat a month without dieting or exercising? Well it's true! You can actually burn fat at the rate of a pound a day or more, but that would not be advisable. This chemical has been clinically tested and proven to burn fat at this rate per day. It has been clinically proven to be virtually harmless to the human body, when used correctly. The only exceptions are the two known allergic reactions that are fairly rare and of course overdosing is harmful as with any substance. That's it!

It gets better too! It works for virtually *everyone* and many clinicians describe its effects on the human body as exactly the same as those that accompany exercise. That's right, you can actually take a pill and burn off one half pound of fat a day in pretty much the same way as if you were exercising, without dieting or exercise.

There is more good news! This substance is actually better than exercise in a couple of ways. There is at least one study done in recent times in which a doctor shows that weight lost with this substance

> "This substance is actually better than exercise!"

stays off easier than with dieting and exercise. That's right, you won't have the same difficulty with keeping the lost weight off as with other weight loss methods! Another plus is that there is no muscle wasting. Muscle wasting is losing muscle along with fat. Diet and exercise *do cause* muscle wasting. This stuff actually *fights* muscle wasting. When you lose ten pounds with this stuff, it is almost *entirely* fat. There is even more good news that I will cover later on in this book.

My book is about making this chemical known, but it is also about revealing the sad reality, that is just as important a part of the truth of this chemical's story. You see, at one time this substance was a legal prescription and non-prescription medicine in the United States of America. Hard to believe, I know. The FDA banned it a very long time ago for a ridiculous excuse of a reason. In my opinion, special interest and greed are the real motivations that are keeping it from legal prescription use by the American people. How can this be?

Fact: Each year 652,091 people die from heart attack and 143,579 die from stroke.
http://www.cdc.gov/nchs/FASTATS/deaths.htm

You are rightly thinking that a drug that can do what you've just read would perhaps be the most important medicine known to man. It would be a dream come true for countless people. I believe, or more precisely, I am absolutely convinced, that these things are true about this chemical.

My book will prove everything I have just stated beyond any reasonable doubt. Please keep an open mind, because how this book fares will decide whether the American public has the power to use this substance to rid it itself of the scourge of obesity and excess fat forever. There are extremely powerful industries, including perhaps the largest industry in this country, that will do everything in their power to stop this chemical from being made legal.

By publishing this book, I have put myself in a somewhat risky position by being a financial threat to these interest groups to the tune of hundreds of billions of dollars in lost profits. For example, it is almost certain that one large multibillion-dollar industry would basically evaporate into thin air, in a very short time, if this chemical were allowed as a prescription drug again. I cover this scenario in more detail later in the book.

I am willing to accept the obvious risks involved with this endeavor in the hope, however remote, that the American People will benefit from this chemical becoming a legal prescription drug again. The knowledge that hundreds of millions of Americans and countless other people around the world could be both healthier and happier because they would become quickly and easily thin, is something I could not walk away from.

The following four paragraphs are a list of assertions; some not yet stated above, that this book will show to be true and reasonable:

- There is a chemical, that was once a prescription medicine in the United States. It is the most effective fat reduction therapy known and has been clinically proven to reduce fat faster than any other non-surgical therapy known (liposuction is the one possible exception). It burns off fat for everyone that uses it without exception. Many people have used it to burn up to a pound (or more) of fat a day. Not a combination of fat, muscle and water weight like almost any other weight loss method, including diet and exercise, but almost pure fat.

- This chemical's existence is, for the most part, unknown to the American public, primarily because it was banned by the FDA for use as a fat reduction therapy, not long before the USA entered the Second World War. This ban came after years of successful use by several hundred thousand Americans as a prescription and over the counter medicine to reduce fat. Whatever the real motivation for this ban was, it has been an incalculable tragedy. That this ban continues is inexcusable, unjust and is a medical and societal tragedy of overwhelming proportions.

- This chemical is so perfectly suited for fat reduction that if it were returned to use as a prescription medicine for fat reduction, virtually all other existing therapies for that purpose would become obsolete. Given the role greed and special interests play in our political system there is little chance it will ever be returned to its legal status as a prescription medicine. To compound the problem, misinformation about this chemical is so pervasive and so negative that it is all but impossible for an individual, who happened to learn of its existence, to see the truth about it clearly enough to be willing to use it.

- This truth, that is so obscured, is that this chemical in addition to its nonpareil effectiveness, is truly harmless, in that it does no damage to humans and has no serious side effects* if not overdosed. Furthermore, it is so perfectly suited for fat reduction therapy, both from a standpoint of its effectiveness and its harmlessness to the human body, that it has been described in clinical reports as having the same effect on the body as exercise. This chemical acts on the body to burn fat with such simple effectiveness, it would be hard to think of a realistic way to improve its mode of action, efficiency, efficacy, flexibility or benignity. It has the additional advantage of being dirt cheap as a bulk powder.

"the solution to the single greatest health crisis in America"

It is the position of the author, that this book does indeed prove the above four propositions to be true and factual and consequently the central theses to be true: that America is indeed being deprived of a substance, that would be the solution to the single greatest health crisis in America.

*There are two relatively rare "allergic reactions" that are discussed extensively throughout this book

A Brief Analogy

Until the middle of the 20th century, infections like staph and strep were a terrible scourge that often took several young children from each family as illness swept through neighborhoods and cities, leaving a trail of death and devastation. Rather than use statistics to illustrate this harsh reality, that our ancestors endured, I will relate my grandmother's description of her own experience and the experience of her family and the families in her neighborhood, when she was a child.

In the first decade of the last century my grandmother's parents lost one child to infection as an infant. She remembered seeing her baby sister's casket in the small family living room. She was five years old at the time. She told me her family was actually the luckiest in her neighborhood. Every other family had lost multiple children. Many families had more dead than living children and one family had lost all six of their children to disease and infection.

This is what life was like without antibiotics. Most of those children had tragically succumbed to bacterial or viral infection only because antibiotics had not yet been discovered. Parents were virtually defenseless. Whatever they could do was often insufficient to save their children. They could only watch desperately as their children faded and died, when a bottle of penicillin would have made the situation little more than an inconvenience. Fast forward to today, a trip to the doctor and pharmacist, then a few days of missed school. Quite a contrast to one or several of your children dying, wouldn't you say?

You might be wondering what this has to do with a miracle fat loss chemical. Well, imagine for a moment that the FDA had banned antibiotics back in the 1950s. Let's say the reason they banned them was for some relatively minor side effect that affected less than 1% of those who took it, and that side effect could be effectively averted, even for the few who were affected. Since that time, the very existence of antibiotics had become virtually unknown to the American public. The little public information available consisted of a mythology about antibiotics claiming that they were incredibly dangerous and harsh. Furthermore, your research of the clinical studies and medical prescription history during the period that antibiotics were legal did not support this negative hype in any way. As a matter of fact, your research told you, beyond any shadow of a doubt, that antibiotics would save countless lives and avert terrible suffering and that though a small minority were allergic to them, antibiotics were in no way detrimental to people's health, if used properly.

Perhaps, you see the point I am making with this analogy. While it is a stretch to believe this could have happened with antibiotics, it did happen with the chemical that is the subject of this book. For whatever reason, a terrible injustice has been done to the American public, by its government. Worse still, there is almost no possibility of the FDA reversing its decision.

This is just as tragic as if antibiotics had been wrongly kept from us. Perhaps it is even more tragic, considering the fact that a far greater number of people are afflicted with health problems related to obesity than any other cause. Obesity is the number one health problem by far in this US. This makes it all the more pressing that this chemical is once again a prescription medicine.

> "This is just as tragic as if antibiotics had been wrongly kept from us"

This situation needs to be rectified. Providence has provided us with an effective weapon to combat dangerous microbes and likewise has given us an effective weapon to combat obesity. This book is intended to achieve two things: First, to convince the American people of the truth about this substance, so that it can return to its proper status as a prescription medicine. Secondly, its purpose is to make people in every corner of the world aware of this substance, so they can take advantage of it.

Description and History

Extra body fat is a chronic scourge of overwhelming proportions afflicting modern humanity. From that frustratingly stubborn extra 10 pounds, to clinical obesity, excess body fat undermines the health and happiness of billions of people around the world.

There are ways to combat excess fat, from diet and exercise, to prescription medicines to surgical procedures, but still the problem remains, and is getting worse. There is a chemical compound that could do more to free the world of this scourge, than all other weight loss therapies combined: That chemical is 2,4 Dinitrophenal, better known as DNP.

DNP has been in existence since the 1800s. It is a manufactured chemical and does not occur naturally. It is a crystalline solid, yellow in color, and has a distinct odor that is described as musty and sweet and has been compared to the smell of Rosewood or Cherry Wood.

It dissolves moderately well in water, not very well in cold water. It stains everything it touches with a yellow tint. The stains are very hard to remove. It is easily airborne and subsequently inhaled. It can be combined with other chemicals, for a variety of industrial uses.

Various Commercial Industrial Uses

One of DNP's early uses was in the manufacturing of explosives in France. Subsequent uses have included its use as wood preservative, an insecticide, a dye and in the film developing process. Today it is primarily used in manufacturing and various types of scientific research.

In the early 1900s it was found to cause dramatic weight loss in workers continuously exposed to large concentrations of it. This eventually led to experimentation with animals. The following collection of quotes from *Dr. Horner's valuable analyses* circa 1942, provides some of the findings of animal studies led by Drs. Cutting and Tainer of Stanford University Medical Clinics.

> *"In 1931, Tainter and Cutting and their associates began an elaborate series of independent studies on the pharmacology of dinitrophenol...Pulse rate and blood-pressure were not raised...The increased metabolism was primarily at the expense of fats and carbohydrates...The fatal dose for various species was determined at 20 to 30 mg. per kilogram of body weight...In experimental animals death resulted from direct circulatory depression, high fever, acidosis, and anoxemia. Tainter and Cutting were unable to find any significant damage to important organs of dogs given daily, just short of fatal, doses of dinitrophenol for periods of six months."*[1]

In addition to the fact that DNP did not damage organs, even when severely overdosed in these experiments confirmed what had been deduced from the experience with accidental human exposure. DNP was found to be an extremely efficient fat burner through an increase in the basal metabolic rate.

Clinical, Prescription and Popular Therapeutic Use

Following the discoveries from clinical studies of animals, Drs. Cutting and Tainter of Stanford University, then did a series of controlled clinical studies and released clinical research papers, in 1933, concluding that DNP caused dramatic weight loss through fat reduction. This was the first clinical report to show DNP to have a human therapeutic application. This excerpt from Dr. Horner's classic 1942 document gives some of the findings from human testing:

> "In human beings "the action of dinitrophenol agreed closely with that observed in animals in equivalent doses. In July, 1933, Cutting, Mehrtens and Tainter" reported that nine patients had been given from 3 to 5 hundred mg. of the drug daily for periods of from one to ten weeks. In six of these the metabolic rate was repeatedly determined and was found to be maintained at an average of 40 per cent. above normal. All these subjects lost weight without dietary restrictions. Changes in temperature, pulse rate, and respiration were not observed, although the amount of perspiration was increased. No undesirable symptoms were encountered, and the patients stated that they felt better and were more active than before taking the drug."[2]

DNP immediately became a medicine prescribed by physicians for fat reduction. Over the course of the next year, clinical studies were undertaken in countries around the world including: Canada, Great Britain, France, Sweden, Italy, and Australia. DNP's growth in popularity in the US as a prescription medicine, in that same year, was staggering. At the Stanford University's Clinics alone, approximately 4,500 patients were treated an average of 3 months each. It was estimated by the doctors at Stanford that over 100,000 Americans were treated that same year by prescription use of DNP around the country.

At the same time, its use as a non-prescription medicine was exploding. The number of companies that sold DNP multiplied at a spectacular rate. There were already more than 20 within this first year. It was sold under a variety of names such as Slim, Dinitrenal,

Nitraphen, Dinitrole Redusols and Formula 17, sometimes with DNP as the sole ingredient and sometimes as a concoction comprised of DNP and other substances. There was no real regulation of this use, because at that time the FDA did not possess the same range of regulatory powers it does today.

In 1934, Drs. Cutting and Tainter produced a report[1] covering the results of their combined clinical studies, their experience with prescription use at the Stanford clinics, and the estimated 100,000 Americans that were prescribed DNP around the country by other doctors. This report remains the definitive critical analyses of human therapeutic use of DNP and I quote from it more than any other single source in this book. (This report can be found in its complete form in the clinical studies section of this book.)

> **FACT: Obesity increases the risk of Type 2 Diabetes and several types of cancer.**
> http://www.cdc.gov/nccdphp/dnpa/obesity/

DNP was on the market, both as a prescription and non-prescription drug, until 1938, when the FDA banned it. The Food, Drug and Cosmetic act of 1938 was a precedent setting piece of legislation, in which the FDA exercised a vast new array of regulatory powers. DNP was among the casualties of this sweeping regulatory act. The official reason the FDA gave for its ban on DNP was that it was thought to cause cataracts in one percent of women who used it. After the FDA imposed ban on DNP, it slowly declined from the American public's consciousness.

During this whole five-year period of legal public use, conservatively estimated at over 500,000 patients, Doctor Horner points out that there was a total of 9 reported deaths[1] mostly from overdose. Strangely, there were three deaths from a rare blood disorder that DNP was clinically shown not to cause, included in these nine deaths.

This is an extremely low occurrence of accidental overdose, compared to many prescription drugs today. In other words, DNP has an exceptionally low risk of fatal overdose, compared to a present day prescription medications like Vicodin®. It did have a brief resurgence in the 1980's, when Dr. Bachinsky opened a chain of clinics in Texas that used DNP to bring about weight loss. By the time the FDA shut the operation down, he had treated more than 14,000 patients. There were no deaths and no injuries claimed or lawsuits pursued by the clients of Dr. Bachinsky that I have been able to find.

CHAPTER TWO

Effectiveness as a Fat Reduction Therapy

DNP is the most effective fat burner known. It has been clinically documented to burn amazing amounts of fat. Many modern day users report losing a pound of pure fat a day, some have lost even more. DNP's mode of burning fat is, biochemically speaking, identical to exercise. Many people make this comparison. To doctors

> "the most effective fat burner known"

and clinicians personally familiar with its therapeutic effects, this comparison of DNP's effects on the body to exercise is axiomatic. It is even found in clinical studies. For example:

> *"As for physical exercise, it seems to act exactly like dinitro therapy. Marcowitz, in his communication to the Academy of Medicine of Toronto on October 9, 1934, based on 90 cases of obesity, having followed this treatment during a period of 16 months, concludes that its action may be succinctly described in saying that the effects on the organism are similar to those of physical exercises."*[3]

> "Even diet and exercise are not nearly as consistently effective."

DNP increases the body's basal metabolic rate. That is the rate at which the body expends energy (burns fat), while at rest. The body does not have a negative feedback mechanism to limit this metabolic increase. Consequently, DNP works for almost *everyone* with an amazing and inexorable efficiency. Even diet and exercise are not nearly as consistently effective. The body does have ways of adjusting to and so thwarting, many people's attempts to burn off fat in this manner. When it comes to diet and exercise, what works for one person does not work nearly as well for another. This is not the case with DNP, it always works its fat burning magic.

Every 100 milligrams of DNP causes an average eleven percent increase in the basal metabolic rate (the rate the body uses energy at complete rest). From everything I've read in studies and modern underground use, this translates to roughly one tenth of a pound of fat burned every 24 hours. Drs. Cutting and Tainter of

> **"this translates to roughly one tenth of a pound of fat burned every 24 hours"**

Stanford University reported, that a fifty percent increase could be safely maintained for extended periods (three months was an average treatment duration). That is an astounding rate; over one half pound of fat a day. In this, Tainter and Cutting led Stanford University study (one of their earlier ones), described below, by Dr. Horner, they used smaller doses with excellent results. These good results were in spite of the fact, that about half of these patients were not responding to any other therapy and were considered to be very difficult cases.

"In November, 1933, Tainter, Stockton, and Cutting published a progress report covering 113 consecutive, unselected cases of obesity treated by dinitrophenol. The patients consisted of 98 females and 15 males. About one half of the cases had received previous thyroid administration and had undergone dietary regimens until no further weight loss was effected, hence they represented the more unresponsive types of obesity.

The treatment was successful in 101 (89.4 per cent.) cases. An average loss of weight of between two and three pounds (0.9 to 1.3 kg.) a week was obtained by an average daily dose of 0.3 gm. The weight loss was shown by measurements to be predominantly from hips and abdomen. Those patients who were not on special diets at the beginning of the treatment were allowed to eat their regular fare without restrictions.

Individuals who had taken the drug continuously for four months showed no demonstrable evidence of cumulative or toxic effects. Certain side actions were observed in others;"[1]

Dosing will be covered in greater detail in the Dosing section in part two of this book. The excerpt from a relatively modern study[4] below shows how effective DNP can be at safe and comfortable doses.

The test subjects of this study, two men and one woman, ingested DNP daily, for an average of roughly nine months.

Here are the numbers for the woman: After 241 days of DNP treatment, she had gone from 208 pounds to 135 pounds. This is a loss of 73 pounds, without a low calorie diet and no exercise in 8 months, at comfortably low doses of DNP. The average weight lost between the three subjects is roughly nine pounds a month and none of the weight was regained afterward, for a subsequent period of months that the subjects were monitored. Compare that to diet and exercise, where people generally regain the lost weight and then gain some additional weight too.

Here is the female subject's chart progress:

TABLE 1

Day	Weight (lbs)
1	208 1/2
19	202 1/2
35	196 1/2
49	189 1/2
69	184
92	175
113	167
134	160
155	152 1/2
180	148
206	146
241	135

Here are the two men's charts:

TABLE 2

Day	Weight (lbs)
1	255
14	241
30	232
44	227
65	220
76	214
97	208
125	203
153	197 3/4
181	193
209	189
279	178
321	167

TABLE 3

Day	Weight (lbs)
1	354
24	333
38	314
59	317
80	297 1/4
101	288
122	275
143	260 1/2
164	254
185	243 1/2
206	246
227	235 1/2
248	234
269	229
290	222

The statistics for the results of the two men treated with DNP in the study are as follows: The first man lost 88 pounds in 321 days. This man started with a lower dosing schedule than the lady in the study, but was subsequently given the same doses after 59 days. The third test subject lost 130 pounds in 222 days. In this study, an additional compound was used along with DNP, but the rate of fat loss does not differ from other studies done decades before this one was done.

CHAPTER THREE

Mode of Action on the Human Metabolism

All of the cells in the human body use a basic form of energy to perform their various functions. This energy is called ATP and the cells keep a reserve of it available at all times. When you exercise, you deplete these ATP reserves. Without ATP your cells cannot function or survive. Fortunately, our bodies have a backup plan to replenish ATP, it burns three readily available energy sources: carbohydrates, fat and protein, but mostly fat. This is why you lose fat when you exercise. You are burning ATP and your body replenishes it by burning up your fat reserves.

DNP makes the conversion to ATP less efficient by a process that hijacks the ATP conversion process, turning it to energy that is burnt off. This in turn depletes your ATP, so your body is forced to burn fat to make up for the shortfall. Both

> **"its symptoms and side effects are essentially the same as exercise."**

exercise and DNP burn fat as a consequence of ATP depletion. For this reason and the fact that DNP has a simple, direct and entirely physiological effect at a cellular level, DNP's symptoms and side effects are essentially the same as exercise.

Refer to the box on the next page for a more technical, scientific description of DNPs mechanism of basal metabolic increase.

DNP's action is at a cellular level and entirely physiological. It serves as a protonophore passing the Mitochondrial Membrane protonated returning as an anion. This repeating cycle causes an increase in the proton conductance of the Mitochondria subsequently uncoupling oxidative phosphorylation causing inefficiency in the production of Adenosine triphosphate (ATP). Some of the energy that normally accompanies cellular respiration is partially thrown off as excess heat. The basal metabolic rate increases to make up for the shortfall brought on by the inefficient loss of energy. This means increased fat burning to replenish ATP. This effect is increased on a dose dependant basis. [5,6,7]

CHAPTER FOUR

A Safe and Harmless Medicine
(when used properly, as with any Drug)

> **"there is no limit to how high it can drive your fat burning metabolism!"**

DNP's fat burning is simply dose dependant. Consume more DNP, burn more fat. But this feature has another side. Because the body has no mechanism to limit the metabolic increase effect of DNP, there is no limit to how high it can drive your fat burning metabolism. To put it bluntly, if you take too much DNP, you can kill yourself from overheating and or dehydration. The fact that you can fatally overdose on practically every prescription medicine (or for that matter, any substance humans can otherwise safely ingest) is common knowledge. For instance, if you are given a prescription for Vicodin® to alleviate pain, most likely there is enough Hydrchodone in the bottle to kill you. According to the FDA, as little as eight pills can be lethal. Your health and even your life depend on your following dosing instructions.

The essential difference between the two is that the DNP is dangerous, because it can overly increase your metabolism and Vicodin® is dangerous because it can overly suppress it. But the important thing to note here, is that virtually anything that can be orally consumed safely, can also be overdosed to injury or fatality. Therefore, it is completely ridiculous to call DNP dangerously unacceptable as a medicine simply because it can be overdosed. This would mean virtually every medicine should be illegal.

DNP does no direct serious harm to the body. Multiple clinical studies have proven this. There is also immense clinical experience with prescription and non-prescription use of DNP. It does have side effects, and some people can have allergic reactions. The good thing is that the side effects are for the most part, the same ones that come with the fat burning process of aerobic exercise. For example: overheating, dehydration, exhaustion etc. can, for the most part, be countered with the same protocols used for exercise. These protocols are discussed in detail in part two of this book.

A good way to conceptualize the cause of virtually all of the side effects of DNP is to understand that they are caused by heat resulting from increased fat burning, not some direct chemical action on the body. DNP is not hurting the user's body, rather through a very basic physiological process at the cellular level, it is causing the body to burn fat so efficiently, that heat is produced just like when you exercise. The difference is that the heat can be raised much higher with DNP than it can be with exercise.

> **"virtually all of the side effects... are caused by heat resulting from increased fat burning; not some chemical action on the body."**

DNP has the same effects on the body as exercise through ATP depletion and the subsequent rise in the basal metabolic rate. The increased fat burning is a heat generating process. The side effects from exercise and DNP ingestion such as sweating, excess warmth, etc. are due to this increased fat burning generated heat. The feeling of exhaustion shared by DNP therapy and exercise is an exception; rather than being caused by heat it is caused by the energy depletion itself, that is also common to both.

DNP	Stage	Exercise
Ingest DNP	1	Aerobic Exercise
ATP Depletion	2	ATP Depletion
Exhaustion, Lethargy	3	Exhaustion, Lethargy
Increased Metabolic Quotient	4	Increased Metabolic Quotient
Fat Burning Induced Heat Increase	5	Fat Burning Induced Heat Increase
Heat Related Side Effects (Sweating, Dehydration etc.)	6	Heat Related Side Effects (Sweating, Dehydration etc.)

A person cannot exercise long enough or with sufficient intensity to cause the same degree of fat burning induced heat that extremely high doses of DNP can cause. This is good news for two reasons. DNP always works its fat burning magic with inexorable efficiency and the greater the dose the greater the fat burning. Consequently, DNP can burn fat at a higher rate than anything else known. The other good thing is since DNP's fat burning effect is dose dependent, the fat burning induced heat can be kept at safe and tolerable levels with lower dosing. Even at very safe and tolerable heat levels, DNP still burns fat off the user's body faster than any other known drug or chemical. This quote, from Drs. Cutting and Tainter, shows that not only these two doctors, but other clinicians and doctors also found that DNP is effective at safe and comfortable levels.

" In a preliminary report on the loss of body weight in obese individuals it was stated that losses of 2 to 3 pounds a week could be obtained with doses of dinitrophenol which were well tolerated. Three other groups of workers have confirmed this result in smaller groups of patients, and it is now a common experience with many practicing physicians. "[2]

The FDA is obscuring this truth, in all of their official proclamations, by ignoring this and sometimes even implying the opposite!

It is generally considered safe to increase your basal metabolic rate by about 50%. DNP has been shown to increase the human thermogenic fat burning process by this percentage or more. As you will read later on, increasing your metabolism this much can be an uncomfortable and sweaty ordeal. But the good news is that DNP is effective at much lower doses that are neither unsafe nor uncomfortable.

Fact: A 2005 CDC Study found that 33.3% of American men are obese and 35.3% women are obese.
http://www.cdc.gov/nccdphp/dnpa/obesity/

An increase of 10 to 40% of the basal metabolic rate will still burn fat more effectively than any other weight reduction substance. According to many clinicians and other DNP experts, this is a very safe and comfortable rate. Each increase of the basal metabolic rate by 10% has the effect of burning roughly one tenth of a pound of fat a day. So an increase of 30% is three tenths or nearly one third of a pound of fat burned a day.

It should be noted here, that although the fat burning process produces a lot of heat, this heat is radiated away from the body. Your body temperature at normal therapeutic levels of DNP can go up one or two degrees. The larger concern is not so much with body temperature as it is with dehydration. It cannot be overly stressed how

34

important proper hydration (mostly drinking a lot of water) is when on DNP, especially at higher doses. Since DNP's fat burning rate is dose dependent, its safe use is entirely in the control of the user. The side effects and necessary precautions at higher doses become lessened to almost nonexistent at lower doses and these lower doses are still extremely effective for fast weight loss.

At just a ten percent increase, or just one tenth of a pound a day of fat burned off, a normal person in usual conditions would not notice any side effects. If it was extremely hot outside and the person was jogging, they might notice some of these side effects. Now, there are several fat burning substances that do increase fat burning in a similar way. None of them can increase the metabolic rate or burn fat at close to the rate that DNP does. Ephedrine is one example. It only raises the metabolism by three percent at most and it does have a many negative side effects.

CHAPTER FIVE

Don't Take My Word for it, Listen to the Experts

Here are the words of the top DNP experts. These are the words of the medical doctors who worked as clinicians at some of the most prestigious clinics in the world studying DNP's effects on humans for years:

> **"It acts on the body like exercise. Not poison, not deadly, not even harsh."**

It acts on the body like exercise. Not poison, not deadly, not even harsh.

"As for physical exercise, it seems to act exactly like dinitro therapy. Marcowitz, in his communication to the Academy of Medicine of Toronto on October 9, 1934, based on 90 cases of obesity, having followed this treatment during a period of 16 months, concludes that its action may be succinctly described in saying that the effects on the organism are similar to those of physical exercises."[3]

There will be an outcry that I call DNP "benign," meaning not harmful. That is exactly the concept that the next statement conveys. It clearly states, DNP does not affect or interfere with the body's functions or hurt its major organs and then states flatly that this is a main reason for using it for fat reduction therapy. Hmmm.... nothing here about DNP being poisonous, deadly or harsh:

"This innocuity for the principal visceral functions is without doubt one of the main reasons for the distribution of this therapy."[3]

An animal study showed, when lethal doses of DNP were administered to rats there was no other toxicity found and no abnormities.[8]

Here is an excerpt from Dr. Horner's 1942 document referring to the Stanford University clinicians, also finding that DNP does no harm to organs even when severely overdosed! You can't say that about very many drugs!!!

"In 1931, Tainter and Cutting and their associates began an elaborate series of independent studies on the pharmacology of dinitrophenol...Pulse rate and blood-pressure were not raised...The increased metabolism was primarily at the expense of fats and carbohydrates...The fatal dose for various species was determined at 20 to 30 mg. per kilogram of body weight...In experimental animals death resulted from direct circulatory depression, high fever, acidosis, and anoxemia. Tainter and Cutting were unable to find any significant damage to important organs of dogs given daily,just short of fatal, doses of dinitrophenol for periods of six months"[1]

That was testing on dogs, Dr. Horner also points out that Drs. Cutting and Tainter of Stanford University clinics, found that DNP did not harm humans either. Also, that it was extremely effective:

"the action of dinitrophenol agreed closely with that observed in animals in equivalent doses. In July, 1933, Cutting, Mehrtens and Tainter"[9] reported that nine patients had been given from 3 to 5 mg. per kilogram of the drug daily for periods of from one to ten weeks. In six of these the metabolic rate was repeatedly determined and was found to be maintained at an average of 40 per cent. above normal. All these subjects

lost weight without dietary restrictions. Changes in temperature, pulse rate, and respiration were not observed, although the amount of perspiration was increased. **No undesirable symptoms were encountered, and the patients stated that they felt better and were more active than before taking the drug.** *"[2](emphasis added)*

This report shows no harmful effects on humans:

"A preliminary report is made of the metabolic and therapeutic effects of 2:4 dinitrophenol and 3:5 dinitro-ortho-cresol administered consecutively to 10 schizophrenic patients. Both drugs caused increase in the rate of oxygen consumption with various other metabolic effects indicative of increased oxidative efficiency. The ortho-cresol proved to be the more potent but showed the property of causing discoloration of the skin and scleræ.

The therapeutic results were indeterminate.

Aside from discoloration of the integument by the ortho-cresol neither drug, within the limits of dosage used, caused any perceptible harmful effects."[9]

I have proven that DNP doesn't hurt the body in general, Let's break it down organ system-by-system:

Liver

There are many quotes out there by various government "authorities" about DNP *possibly* harming the liver. Here is one of the premier clinical DNP experts, quoting three of the top clinical experts that "beyond a doubt" the liver is not damaged by DNP treatment.

Tainter, Stockton and Cutting have reported a series of cases in which one had measured the plasma bile index and determined the test of Van de Bergh. Their analyses demonstrate, beyond a doubt, that the <u>liver</u> does not suffer any damage in the course of dinitro treatment. [3]

Ooops, so much for the bad liver claims though, the anti-DNP diatribe will no doubt continue to occasionally include liver damage claims. After all, they have done so in the face of this clinical evidence for decades. You know what they have to base these liver damage accusations on? It was at one time surmised that it might hurt the liver because of its having some vague similarities to another compound that did damage the liver. Also, since DNP is a yellow dye and can cause a yellow tint, it was once thought that it might hurt the liver because the yellow tint was mistaken for jaundice.

> **FACT: Extra weight increases changes of Coronary heart disease.**
> http://www.cdc.gov/nccdphp/dnpa/obesity/

Why do critics still say DNP might damage or does damage the liver? They make these claims because they have nothing substantial, at least nothing that comes close to a reason to ban DNP. The FDA sanctions many drugs that do injure the liver, Lipitor® and Vicodin® among them. Why do they sanction these drugs? They do it partly because those drugs have sufficient benefits to offset the liver damage.

DNP has the best offsetting benefits of any pharmaceutical substance, even if it did do some damage. Even though DNP is clinically proven to not hurt the liver, it does have one side effect that is unacceptable: It is deadly to the weight loss industry and would do tremendous damage to the profits of the medical industry. These are two side effects, that will not be tolerated by their attack dog, the FDA.

They just can't be published as the decisive reasons for banning it, hence the mud at the wall, vague mixture of half-truths is the modus opporendi of the FDA and its parrots.

Kidneys

Experimental studies on animals do not show toxic effects of dinitrophenol on the kidney (Taitner, Cutting, Wood and Proescher). Anatomical-pathological examinations of animals, even those which died from a massive dose of dinitrophenol, do not reveal any important anatomical changes, except a small degree of cytolysis. Clinical documents are not abundant, but, on the whole, do not seem to demonstrate that dinitrophenol is toxic for the kidneys.[3]

Cardiovascular System

Dinitrophenol is remarkable for its absence of effect on the cardio-vascular system. Even when the basal metabolism is found elevated to significant levels, there is no change in the rhythm of the pulse (Rosenblum). On this point, dinitrophenol differs from all the other metabolic accelerants known. It is an observation that all the clinicians, today, have had occasion to make.[3]

All the clinicians know that, contrary to thyroxine, dinitrophenol is absolutely devoid of toxicity for the heart. The research of Professor Loeper and of his students has demonstrated the physiological and clinical importance of myocardiac glycogen. Extensive studies by P.N. Taussig have shown that dinitrophenol does not reduce cardiac glycogen at all and that, on this point, it differs completely from thyroxine.[3]

Gastrointestinal

As to claims that DNP is hard on the stomach, (which can often be found sprinkled in every type of dire warning, including that it is poisonous, for this very reason):

"The claim that this drug is a severe irritant to the gastrointestinal tract of patients is unwarranted for doses of therapeutic range, according to our experience and to that of large numbers of physicians prescribing it."

Not cancer causing but cancer curing.

DNP fights breast cancer effectively. This study shows that it blocks and fights cancerous cells, but has no effect on healthy cells.

"Two membrane-permeable and RNase-resistant antisense poly-2'-O-(2,4-dinitrophenyl)-oligoribonucleotides (poly-DNP-RNAs) have been synthesized as inhibitors of human breast cancerâ€¦fluorescence assay indicates that the targeted antisense inhibition by poly-DNP-RNAs leads to apoptosis of SK- Br-3 cells but does not affect nontumorigenic MCF-10A cells. The control poly-DNP-RNAs with random or sense nucleotide sequence are completely inactive." [10]

One study found that DNP slowed tumor growth by inhibiting their respiration by up to 25%.[11] Another study discovered that DNP caused melanoma cells to self-destruct, but healthy cells remain unaffected.[12]

Yet another study revealed DNP as an effective therapy for inhibiting melanoma (skin cancer). This study deals with oxygenation increase and its acute effect on the cancerous cells only.[13]

Looks like the medical industry's bottom line might have more to fear from DNP than just weight loss. In Part Two of this book you can find the definitive clinical report done on human therapeutic use of DNP.

I have quoted heavily from both of these reports. The one by Dr. Bell is of particular interest, as it was written right after DNP was banned in the USA. He wrote this document to defend DNP as a safe, effective and indispensable therapy for human fat reduction.

CHAPTER SIX

My Personal Experience with this Substance

When I first read of DNP in the body builder forums on the web, I found a pretty dark picture. The more I read though, the more I noticed that there was really no substance to all of the negativity. The only real complaint anyone who had actually used DNP had was that if he or she took really large doses of DNP, he or she got exaggerated symptoms of working out too hard. Eventually, I came across a few people who had done reasonable doses and had little to no side effects at all. No one who used it ever claimed any damage of any kind and many had been using very high doses for years.

A few people had even started to see this truth and mention it. But you have to understand, safety and caution in using the various substances they use, is paramount with body builders in these forums. They tend to warn people in the strongest possible terms against any kind of abuse of any substance, that is part of their sport. A few people who had enough personal exposure to DNP pointed out that it was safe, and not at all harsh when used at the proper dosages. Some of these people pointed out that the side effects were all the same ones that accompany aerobic exercise and completely dose dependant.

I had read bits and pieces from a couple of human clinical studies, and they all supported the safety and efficacy of DNP. I decided that I would try it myself, provided I could find no real health risks after making a serious effort to do so.

After countless dozens, if not hundreds, of hours of research, I found nothing to support the negative hype. Sure there was the danger of overdosing, but every safe substance shares that attribute with DNP. There were the two allergic side effects, but both were rare allergic reactions and every other safe substance has people that are allergic to it . As a result of my extensive study, I knew that neither of these posed an issue to me.

What I did notice is that DNP actually has less effect on the various systems and tissues of the body than any legal drug I could think of, including Tylenol. This is exactly what the clinicians, who had done very extensive human clinical studies, said about DNP; that it really doesn't affect the body other than at the cellular level. It made ATP production less efficient, through an elegantly simple process, but that was it. They even stressed this by pointing out that its effects were purely physiological. In other words, it doesn't affect heart rate or blood pressure and there is no direct effect on the endocrine system. The one exception was a secondary effect. At larger doses, DNP inhibited the conversion of t-4 to t-3, but none of the clinicians thought this was a problem. This attribute actually helps DNP to not cause muscle wasting. This process always returns to normal, with no harmful effects, even after months of use.

Now, it was obvious to me that after five years of legal use by hundreds of thousands of Americans, if there were anything harmful that clinicians had not found, it would have manifested itself in a pattern and been mentioned somewhere from such grand scale use for so many years. Nothing, nada, zip.

> **"after five years of legal use by hundreds of thousands of Americans, if there were anything harmful that clinicians had not found, it would have manifested itself ... Nothing, nada, zip."**

Now, I was already aware of at least two other substances, which have been under various kinds of attack and control for no other conceivable reason than the financial damage they would inflict on the medical and pharmaceutical industries. One of them I consider to be the most valuable medical therapy known (many doctors, scientists and health experts agree), with the exception of DNP. I am researching a companion book to this titled "Illegally Young" that will cover this substance and others. It became obvious to me, that this was the case with DNP. It would almost completely destroy the weight loss industry and it would damage the medical and pharmaceutical industries, to the tune of billions.

Special interest greed was the only conceivable reason for the ban and the vague claims against DNP.

I realized I needed to write a book and tell the truth about DNP. This made it all the more pressing that I try DNP myself. I was not overweight at all, so I decided to only do 10 days worth. I also decided to take fairly strong doses, so I could report the side effects. I settled on 400 mgs of crystalline DNP a day. I started with 200 mg a day for the first two days, just to see how I would react. Also, on the last of the two days, I raised the dose to 600mg, which is generally considered to be a somewhat uncomfortable experience.

> "I raised the dose to 600mg which is generally considered to be a somewhat uncomfortable experience"

I took it in a cold weather situation, I ate an over maintenance calorie diet, (because I wanted to be sure all of my weight loss was from the DNP). For the same reason I did no exercise of any kind, and I drank roughly a gallon of water a day.

The first day I could not really tell anything. The second day, I did just notice some extra warmth, but it was almost imperceptible. By the evening of the third day, I could definitely feel the warmth, but it was not uncomfortable. The next six days were about the same. I remember walking around outside in 30 degree weather in a tee shirt and jeans, and feeling comfortably warm, but even when I was indoors, in a heated room, I was not uncomfortable. I kind of liked feeling warm, actually.

I did sweat a tiny bit, if I was indoors and had too much clothing on, (I normally don't sweat very much at all). I did not really feel lethargic, no more than usual anyway. On the fourth day, I did have one of the possible side effects, I became nauseated. It came after a large spicy Mexican dinner, and lasted about an hour. The occasional nausea is most probably due to electrolyte imbalances brought on by the sweating. Mine could have been caused by the spicy meal, as much as the DNP.

On the last two days the warmth and sweating became more pronounced, but still not bad, though I did feel a little drained on these days as well. I could see where doing 600 mg every day for an extended period could get tedious.

In 10 days, I went from 181 to 175 pounds. I was a little disappointed, because I expected to lose at least eight pounds. I was overeating and doing no exercise of any kind though. At that rate, I would lose eighteen pounds of pure fat a month! Not bad at all.

> **"In 10 days, I went from 181 to 175 pounds"**

I have had no other effects to my health at all. I may use DNP again at some point, just to add to my knowledge and understanding of it.

Between my own experience and all of the other facts I have learned and conveyed in this book, I would not hesitate to advise a friend relative or even one of my children to take DNP, if they needed it. I would just let them know, that to use it legally, that they would have to leave this country.

CHAPTER SEVEN

The Three Real Human Health Concerns
(Overdose and Two Allergic Reactions)

DNP does have the following three real human health concerns: two allergic reactions (cataracts and skin rash) and the possibility of overdose.

In most of the official government documents or statements on DNP, they refer to the overdosing possibility as deadly or poisonous, not mentioning that they are only speaking of overdosing. In addition to this important fact, they also leave out the fact that there are clinically proven, therapeutically safe doses.

In other words, they speak of DNP being deadly or causing death; something any drug can do if overdosed. In addition to this scary and dire warning, they often throw in one or both of the allergic reactions.

> **FACT: Obesity increases the risk of Stroke.**
> http://www.cdc.gov/nccdphp/dnpa/obesity/

In some statements, they add some supposed side effects that they claim DNP causes, that actually have been clinically proven that DNP does not cause. The liver damage claim in the next chapter is an example of one of these inaccuracies.

These official statements always leave the reader ignorant of the fact that many, and as far as I can tell from extensive research of these records, almost all doctors and clinicians who studied DNP, when it was legal, considered it an indispensable and safe medicine. The government's official position is that DNP is a poisonous killer and dangerous contaminant. Clinicians called it the universal fat reduction drug, often pointing out the ways it is safer than other weight reduction drugs. Quite a disparity, don't you think? Anyway, here are the three legitimate health concerns.

1. It is dangerous if overdosed. As has been pointed out already, everything can be overdosed to the point of injury or death, even water; so this attribute is not a knock on DNP relative to anything or everything else, including all legal prescription drugs currently approved by the FDA.

2. Seven percent of patients get an allergic reaction, in the form of a rash, from DNP use. At least 50% of those who get the rash quickly develop a tolerance. In recent times, it has become well known among expert veterans of DNP use, that the rash can be treated successfully with over the counter antihistamines. From what I have read it always works.

3. One in 1000 women who use DNP get cataracts (maybe). This is the FDA's official reason for banning DNP. That pencils out to one tenth of one percent. The FDA conveniently rounds that number up to one percent, by the way. My understanding from my research is that the cataract issue is blown out of proportion to begin with. The European clinicians said it was virtually nonexistent.

There are a number of ways to counteract this side effect now. I can't prove this with clinical studies, but I don't need to. One tenth of one percent, or even one percent is not reason enough to ban a drug, especially one that arguably has greater health benefits than any other. It is a rare allergic reaction.

This is also no reason for men not to be able to use DNP. These supposed DNP induced cataracts occur almost exclusively in female patients. Three men were said to have contracted cataracts during the five years it was legally prescribed. That is out of the at least five hundred thousand people who used DNP. That is less than one in one hundred thousand. I wonder what the rate of occurrence is among men who don't use DNP. It would be strange if it weren't higher, even accounting for age and other factors.

There are also some very strange and questionable facts about the whole cataract issue. First, out of a total of one hundred and seventy seven total cases that were reported during DNP's five-year run as a legal drug, 164 happened in a relatively short period of those five years. Here is Dr. Horner's description;

> "During the summer of 1935 there occurred a sporadic outbreak of cataracts, predominantly in young women, which could have been likened to an epidemic. This began about April, rapidly increased during the summer and fall, and gradually disappeared during 1936-37. Like an epidemic, too, it seemed to point to a common source, namely, dinitrophenol, which was taken for the rapid reduction of body weight. The number of persons who were affected-estimated at more than 164"[3]

It is Dr. Horner, who gives us 177 as the final known count of reported cases in that same 1942 report. It is the definitive synopsis on DNP and cataracts.

The other strange fact, which is also discussed in Dr. Horner's report is that, no clinicians were able to cause cataracts in animals with DNP and many tried really hard, though this in theory could perhaps be an effect that does occur in humans and not in mice.

Add to that the fact, that DNP caused cataracts were almost unknown in Europe, as quoted here:

> "Here we discuss only the case of cataracts, which Horner had said that it occurs in one case in 1000 treatments. At the end of this report we will note the principle bibliographic references concerning the American literature devoted to the subject and which is of a great value, but we wish to emphasize how the European work and especially French are on the other hand still rare and even exceptional...Finally, we emphasize the interest of the work of Vogt on the cataracts caused by dinitrophenol in Switzerland and of G. Ciotola of those caused by alphadinitrophenol in Italy, both published in 1937. The same year, Stein and Crevecoeur pointed out that in their opinion this affectation was, when all is said and done, quite rare if one thinks of the enormous dissemination of dinitro treatment. This was also

the opinion of Andre Mayer, based on the fact that despite the considerable number of intoxications by dintrophenol observed in munitions factories, no cases of cataracts have been noted"[3]

It should also be noted here that Dr. Horner expresses uncertainty, that DNP actually does cause cataracts.

If put together, these facts-

- That 164 out of 177 cases of the cataracts happened in an 18-month period, out of five years total (there is also some evidence that almost all of the 164 happened in California)

- That clinical testing proves DNP does not cause cataracts in animals

- The fact that none of the many workers who were exposed to DNP got cataracts

- That DNP caused cataracts were almost unheard of in Europe

-suggest, that it is more likely that the cataracts were due to some impurity or imperfection in the DNP supply from a particular supplier. But even if it were true that DNP could cause cataracts in one in every three thousand women, (that's what the math really works out to) that would not be a reason to ban such an important drug. The people that are allergic would just not take it, like with any other drug that people are allergic to. There are a lot of drugs that have a more common occurrence of more serious allergic reactions that the FDA approved.

One last thing on this point: Cataract surgery back in the 1930s, was very successful at fixing the problem as Dr. Horner points out. This interesting story related by Jean Sedan (Marseille), from one of the two reported cases in France, is an example of this fact:

"A 32 year old woman weighing 90 kg. (198 pounds) began taking dinitrophenol on February 1st, 1937. She began with 9 to 10 pills daily, each being 30 mg. of DNP. After a week she increased the dose to 12 pills / day (360 mg.). At this dosage she lost 800 grams

per week, or 10 kg. (22 pounds) in three months, without changing her diet. She stopped taking DNP for four months and then began again. So she took 32.4 grams of DNP in the first 90 days and the same amount in the second course. American reports indicated that cataracts had resulted from doses as small as 100 mg. per day for a total of 40 grams.

On June 10th 1938, after several days in a very sunny seaside resort, the patient began to lose vision in her left eye, and on July 12th, the other eye was affected... Indeed, in ending, we repeat the unlikely remark that our second patient made to us upon taking leave following the success of her first operation: "And now, Doctor, do not oppose my taking of dinitrophenol since I no longer risk having cataracts."[3]

This woman was not only successful at repairing her cataract issue with surgery, but she then continued to use DNP. Think about that, she had used DNP for three months at fairly strong doses and was unlucky enough to have the only serious side effect and after dealing with that, she wanted to use DNP again. If it were poisonous or harsh would she want to use it again? Anyway, if they could fix this problem in the 1930's, I would think with today's technology in eye surgery, the rare case could be cured. Not to mention, that Dr. Horner surmised that the problem could be possibly avoided by taking antioxidants like vitamin C.

This is something that many modern day underground use DNP experts claim is a fact.

Under any circumstance, these three health concerns, individually or combined, do not amount to a reason for banning this incredibly effective fat reduction therapy. The one side effect, which cannot be tolerated by the FDA, is what it would do to the weight-loss and medical industries financial bottom lines.

I am not saying there is a conspiracy, in the sense that there is a conscious organized effort over the past eighty years, to keep DNP off the market. While it is of course possible I think that is unlikely.

What I do believe is this, DNP would cause an economic upheaval in a number of ways, if it were reintroduced. As the American public grew in their understanding of DNP's effectiveness and safety, it would not take long before the fat loss industry would basically evaporate. Think about that, a multibillion-dollar industry would be wiped out. Vestiges of that industry that were only partially related to fat loss, like Gyms and certain kinds of health food companies would remain, though not financially unscathed. The rest would be gone. Who would need liposuction, gastric bypass and all those prescription and over the counter "weight loss" drugs that do little or nothing? Good riddance too. It's all just a bunch of snake oil and barbaric surgical profiteering when compared to DNPs simple efficiency.

Now, do you think when faced with DNP, people in that industry won't recognize that financial threat? I don't mean that everyone in those industries is paying nervous attention to DNP. Most don't even know it exists. I mean, to the degree that people in those industries, who play a role in lobbying for and protecting their collective interests, are faced with DNP, they will sense the financial threat. They would rally the industry to react with self-interested motivations, to protect it and their livelihood, by lobbying the government and inciting public opinion against it as dangerous. I believe that has happened to one degree or another a few times since DNP was banned.

Because DNP is illegal, virtually unknown, and has a bad name (unfairly), usually they don't need to do much but occasionally throw a little more mud at the wall, whenever DNP comes up in the news, and it will stick. I am relatively confident that even when they do that they are not fully aware of their misrepresentation. But, they are blinded by self-interest.

Everyone knows the world works this way. Are unions always fair and objective in their negotiations with management? Do they place the welfare of the company or the country in perspective when they negotiate some of their ridiculous demands? No. Do they think they are doing the wrong thing? No. They just see it as their job to negotiate for everything they can. It's a sad fact of human nature. Truth is just the first casualty in the avaricious race to get the upper hand and secure financial advantage. Heck some unions are so greedy they end up destroying the company completely and no one has a job.

By the way, I am not in principle against unions, they are merely the example that came to mind to illustrate this unfortunate aspect of the human social dynamic. Oh well, I am certainly not writing this book to make friends.

CHAPTER EIGHT

Benefit vs. Risk Comparison with FDA Approved Drugs

According to the FDA, their job is to weigh the risks and benefits of each potential drug. They then pass judgment as to whether a drug should be allowed as a legal prescription or over the counter medicine. The FDA listed the rare effect of cataracts and the risk of death by overdose as the reasons DNP is not a legal prescription drug. Death is a red herring, because DNP is not at all deadly, unless overdosed. That is true of every example below and every other legal drug so all they are really saying is this incredibly low occurrence of cataracts in women is almost exclusively the reason DNP was banned. Aside from the fact that such a low occurrence allergic reaction is no reason to ban DNP, it leaves them with absolutely no reason not to allow men to use it. The only reasonable and rather obvious conclusion is that they are protecting the existence of the two industries that lobby them the most. The American people are being robbed of the most valuable medicine known to man because of greed, self-interest and abuse of the power concentrated in the FDA.

> "The American people are being robbed of the most valuable medicine known to man"

The following comparison between the benefits and risks/side effects ratio of DNP and the drugs they *do* allow proves this beyond any reasonable doubt. DNP blows every other method away when this ratio between benefits and risks is the criteria. I promise, if this book is a success, very large and influential industries will publicly proclaim the untrue and overstated risks of DNP. Don't be fooled by that lie. DNP is deadly only in the same sense that every

57

drug the FDA does allow is deadly when overdosed. As a matter of fact Cutting and Tainter point out that the death occurrence ratio to popular and somewhat uncontrolled use was so low, it was "cause for gratification".

DNP

Benefits

- Lowers body fat faster and more efficiently than any other known drug.

- Lowers at the rate of $^1/_3 - \frac{1}{2}$ of a pound of pure fat a day, at clinically proven safe levels, in a manner that has the same effects on the human body as exercise.

- At lower therapeutic doses, DNP has little to no noticeable side effects, while still outperforming any other fat reduction drug by far.

- The advantages to fat reduction are almost countless, but a partial list includes:

    ✓ Lower risk of heart attack

    ✓ Lower risk of stroke

    ✓ Lower cholesterol

    ✓ Lower risk of cancer

    ✓ Lower risk of a plethora of possible health problems with most organs and systems in the body

    ✓ Considerably longer life expectancy

    ✓ Higher self esteem and quality of life

- In other words, DNP has the best overall health benefits and is needed by more people than any drug ever discovered.

- DNP also has the best quality of life benefits of any drug known and is needed for that purpose by more people than any other drug.

Risks

- **Common Side Effects (same as exercise)**

  - ➢ Lethargy

  - ➢ Sweating

  - ➢ Feeling warm

  - ➢ Dehydration

- **Rare Side Effects**

  - ➢ Extremely rare occurrence of cataracts in (women only)

  - ➢ Rash – 7 percent

  - ➢ Headache

  - ➢ Nausea

Lipitor®

Lipitor® is a drug that is meant to lower cholesterol. It works for some, but not all, and is meant to be part of an overall program including diet and exercise. Lipitor® actually has most of the harmful side effects that are wrongfully attributed to DNP by government officialdom. Its' benefits pale in comparison to DNP. Its side effects are both more numerous and serious. The FDA can't possibly give a reasonable explanation that it allows Lipitor® and not DNP.

Benefits

- Lipitor® is meant to lower cholesterol, and does this effectively in some people

Risks

- **Common Side Effects**

    ➢ Headache
    ➢ Constipation
    ➢ Diarrhea
    ➢ Gas
    ➢ Upset stomach and stomach pain
    ➢ Rash
    ➢ Muscle and joint pain

- **Serious Side Effects** –Taken from Lipitor's® own information on their product[15]:

    "LIPITOR® can cause serious side effects. These side effects have happened only to a small number of people. Your doctor can monitor you for them. These side effects usually go away if your dose is lowered or

LIPITOR® is stopped. These serious side effects include:"

> **Muscle problems.** LIPITOR can cause serious muscle problems that can lead to kidney problems, including kidney failure. You have a higher chance for muscle problems if you are taking certain other medicines with LIPITOR.
> **Liver problems.** LIPITOR can cause liver problems. Your doctor may do blood tests to check your liver before you start taking LIPITOR, and while you take it.

Call your doctor right away if you:

> Have muscle problems like weakness, tenderness, or pain that happen without a good reason, especially if you also have a fever or feel more tired than usual
> Have nausea and vomiting
> Pass brown or dark-colored urine
> Feel more tired than usual
> Notice the skin and whites of your eyes become yellow
> Have stomach pain

Who Should NOT Take LIPITOR:

> Women who are pregnant or think they may be pregnant, or may become pregnant. LIPITOR may harm your unborn baby. If you get pregnant, stop taking LIPITOR and call your doctor right away
> Women who are breastfeeding. LIPITOR can pass into your breast milk and may harm your baby
> People with liver problems
> People allergic to LIPITOR or any of its ingredients

Vicodin®

Benefits

- Pain Killer

- Recreation & Relaxation (just kidding)

Risks[16]

- **Adverse Reactions**

The most frequently reported adverse reactions are:

> - lightheadedness,
>
> - dizziness,
>
> - sedation,
>
> - nausea
>
> - vomiting.

These effects seem to be more prominent in ambulatory than in nonambulatory patients and some of these adverse reactions may be alleviated if the patient lies down.

- **Other adverse reactions include:**

Central Nervous System/Psychiatric: Drowsiness, mental clouding, lethargy, impairment of mental and physical performance, anxiety, fear, dysphoria, psychic dependence, mood changes.

Gastrointestinal System: Prolonged administration of hydrocodone bitartrate and acetaminophen elixir may produce constipation.

Genitourinary System: Ureteral spasm, spasm of vesical sphincters, and urinary retention have been reported with opiates.

Respiratory Depression: Hydrocodone bitartrate may produce dose-related respiratory depression by acting directly on the brain stem respiratory centers (see OVERDOSAGE).

Dermatological: Skin rash, pruritus.

The following adverse drug events may be borne in mind as potential effects of acetaminophen: allergic reactions, rash, thrombocytopenia, agranulocytosis.

Potential effects of high dosage are listed in the OVERDOSAGE section.

Infrequently Observed
All adverse events tabulated below are classified as infrequent.

Central Nervous: headache, shaky feeling, tingling, agitation, fainting, fatigue, heavy eyelids, high energy, hot spells, numbness, sluggishness, seizure. Mental confusion, excitement or depression can also occur due to intolerance, particularly in elderly or debilitated patients, or due to overdosage of butalbital.

Autonomic Nervous: dry mouth, hyperhidrosis.

Gastrointestinal: difficulty swallowing, heartburn, flatulence, constipation.

Cardiovascular: tachycardia.

Musculoskeletal: leg pain, muscle fatigue.

Genitourinary: diuresis.

Miscellaneous: prurits, fever, earache, nasal congestion, tinnitus, euphoria, allergic
reactions.

Hydrocodone:
Toxic dose 40 mg
  (8 capsules of hydrocodone bitartrate, butalbital, caffeine, and acetaminophen)

What should I tell my health care provider before I take this medicine?

They need to know if you have any of these conditions:

- glaucoma
- hardening or blockages of the arteries or heart blood vessels
- heart disease or a heart defect
- high blood pressure
- history of alcohol or drug abuse
- history of stroke
- over-active thyroid gland
- psychotic illness, depressed mood, or suicidal thoughts
- recent weight loss
- seizure disorder
- Tourette's syndrome
- an unusual or allergic reaction to dextroamphetamine, other amphetamines, other medicines, foods, dyes, or preservatives
- pregnant or trying to get pregnant
- breast-feeding[16]

Adderall®

Benefits[17]

- Treatment for ADHD

Side effects that you should report to your doctor or health care professional as soon as possible[17]:

•allergic reactions like skin rash, itching or hives, swelling of the face, lips, or tongue
•anxiety, nervousness
•changes in mood or behavior
•chest pain
•fast, irregular heartbeat
•fever, or hot, dry skin
•high blood pressure
•muscle twitching
•uncontrollable head, mouth, neck, arm, or leg movements

Side effects that usually do not require medical attention (report to your doctor or health care professional if they continue or are bothersome):

•difficulty sleeping
•dizziness or light headedness
•headache
•nausea, vomiting
•stomach cramps
•weight loss

This list may not describe all possible side effects.[17]

CHAPTER NINE

Various Negative Claims Analyzed
(Explanation of Specific Examples of Poisonous or Dangerousness Claims)

Watch the pattern. These quotes all share the same attributes. These critics state half-truths, such as DNP is deadly. Then they lump these claims together with a bunch of harmless side effects, which they characterize as also very dangerous or terrible. Sometimes, they throw in one or both of the known allergic reactions, usually failing to mention that they are allergic reactions. Sometimes, for good measure, they will throw in a couple of outright untruths.

> **FACT: Obesity increases the risk of liver and gall bladder disease.**
> CDC Statistic.
> http://www.cdc.gov/nccdphp/d
> nna/obesity/

I call the assertion that DNP is deadly a half-truth, because they fail to mention therapeutic ingestion of DNP is deadly only if overdosed. And that DNP used at normal therapeutic doses is not deadly or even harmful.

Why do they bother to even discuss these rare allergic reactions and overdosing in this way? Because banned substances have official classifications and descriptions and the subject comes up in various contexts and catalogs of information. They repeat the information they find from a previous source to complete the description for whatever their publication purposes are. After all, DNP is both banned and categorized as a poisonous substance. There has to be a reason. So they lay out all the phony dangers for your information and edification. There is no meat to the claims against DNP, because it is not banned for legitimate reasons, just petty bureaucrats repeating the same old meaningless list of vagaries and half-truths. Read below and see for yourself.

This little gem is right from the horse's mouth. It is taken from court documents, regarding the use of DNP.

> *"The use of DNP as a weight loss drug in the 1930s caused numerous deaths and other serious adverse reactions and is one of the incidents that led Congress to enact the Federal Food, Drug, and Cosmetic Act in 1938."*[18]

That's the FDA making things clear for us. Let's look at it this way: How many drugs legally prescribed today, with the FDA's blessing, have "caused numerous deaths and other serious adverse reactions?" For example, how about my favorite whipping boy Vicodin® and all of his dastardly opiate relatives? How many deaths do you think? How much addiction? How many "serious adverse effects"? Well the number of deaths attributed to this class of drugs is off the charts. I have read in several places that they are now the number two cause of accidental death in this country.

Now, don't accuse me of arguing that if one bad class of drugs is legal, it's only fair to allow another. I don't think Vicodin® is bad. As a matter of fact, I like Vicodin®, maybe a little too much. Seriously, what I am saying is that opiate drug related death and destruction is overwhelmingly due to overdosing and other user abuse.

The FDA doesn't bother to point out that this is the only sense in which this is true of DNP's history of therapeutic use. I won't get into the motives and culpability of the person(s) who wrote that statement. It really doesn't matter. Whether they had some sense they were misrepresenting things or not, they were. But if you doubt they were wrong, just read the good doctors and clinicians, who studied DNP. They are quoted throughout this book, and some of their complete reports and papers can be found in the clinical studies section.

The bigger point here is that this is a perfect example of the other claims against DNP. They are almost always vague and often inaccurate. Specific and accurate wouldn't work, as they would not explain the legal status of DNP. Please read the sections that cover the benefits and risks of DNP, if you don't agree. DNP's benefit risk ratio blows away the FDA sanctioned Vicodin,® for instance. (Unless you are already thin and have kidney stones, then you would probably have to give the benefits edge to Vicodin®)

This masterpiece of vague language and convenient characterization is from the EPA.(Environmental Protection Agency):

Non-Cancer: 2,4-Dinitrophenol is a potent uncoupler of oxidative phosphorylation, and may cause methemoglobinemia. Acute exposure orally in humans has resulted in nausea, vomiting, sweating, dizziness, and headache. Chronic oral exposure in humans and animals has resulted in formation of cataracts and skin lesions and has caused effects on the bone marrow, central nervous system, and cardiovascular system. [19]

The United States Environmental Protection Agency (U.S. EPA) has determined that data are inadequate to set a Reference Concentration (RfC) for 2,4-dinitrophenol, but has established an oral Reference Dose (RfD) of 0.002 milligrams per kilogram per day based on cataract formation in humans. The U.S. EPA estimates that consumption of this dose or less, over a lifetime, would not likely result in the occurrence of chronic, non-cancer effects. [19]

No information is available on adverse reproductive or developmental effects of 2,4-dinitrophenol in humans. According to available animal studies, fetal growth inhibition, but no birth defects, were reported in the offspring of animals fed 2,4-dinitrophenol (U.S. EPA, 1994a). [19]

Cancer: No information is available on the carcinogenic effects of 2,4-dinitrophenol in humans. Results from one oral study in mice indicated no tumor formation occurred after six months exposure, and in another study results indicated 2,4-dinitrophenol did not promote tumor development in mice. The International Agency for Research on Cancer and the U.S. EPA have not classified 2,4-dinitrophenol for potential human carcinogenicity. [19]

Well, what a tangled web we weave. If we are to unravel this mess it will have to be one paragraph at a time. The first paragraph is so full of vague and inaccurate statements it will need to be broken down assertion by assertion:

2,4-Dinitrophenol is a potent uncoupler of oxidative phosphorylation, and may cause methemoglobinemia. [19]

No, it doesn't cause *methemoglobinemia*. I researched that condition and its symptoms are shown by Cutting and Tainter to not occur from DNP fat reduction therapy. Read for yourself, in figure 3 at the end of this chapter. I put it there because the quote is rather long and boring. Anyway, the EPA only says here that DNP *"may"* cause it. Boy, they will grasp anything. Just so they could throw in a big scary sounding word, they said it *may* cause something, and they were wrong. Good gosh, the report in which the quote that proves them wrong, is the preeminent and definitive report on DNP from the preeminent experts on it. What the heck do theses government hacks research to write their DNP stuff anyway?

Acute exposure orally in humans has resulted in nausea, vomiting, [19]

"Acute exposure" is quasi-technical terminology in the vernacular of the medical profession. It is used here to mean a kind of concentrated or excessive exposure. Like with anything, if you ingested way too much, you would get nauseated and then throw up. So if that's what the EPA means, it's stupidly obvious as you could do the same with salt or aspirin or practically any other substance. If they are saying that these symptoms are normally caused with standard therapeutic doses, they are being deceptive, to put it politely. Here are the good doctors Cutting and Tainter on this very subject.

> *The claim that this drug is a severe irritant to the gastrointestinal tract of patients is unwarranted for doses of therapeutic range, according to our experience and to that of large numbers of physicians prescribing it.*[2]

To be fair, DNP can cause nausea and or vomiting, but it is an exception. Many medications that most people otherwise tolerate well do occasionally, for whatever reason, cause upset stomachs.

The point is that they have made the claim that DNP will make you sick, lumping this claim together in a list of other supposed dangers. This gives the impression that we are talking about a poisonous chemical, not fit for human consumption, which by the way is exactly what the FDA and EPA say about DNP. The reality is that clinical testing, doctor prescription use and over the counter use prove that this is not the case. To call this quote an overstatement, would be an understatement. It is a misrepresentation of the facts.

> *Acute exposure orally in humans has resulted in...sweating, dizziness, and headache.*[19]

Studies have shown, at the higher therapeutic levels and above these levels DNP does cause sweating, lethargy, and headache. (I say lethargy instead of dizziness because I am pretty sure they meant exhaustion or lethargy instead of dizziness.) At any rate, these symptoms are all due to the rise in the basal metabolic rate. That's increased fat burning, which is the same as the fat burning that accompanies exercise. Actually, to be precise, the relatively rare headache is from dehydration caused by sweating and is alleviated by a glass of water. There is no harm in any of these symptoms.

No clinician, who studied DNP, ever expressed alarm at these side effects. Those clinicians simply pointed out that these effects are the body's normal reaction to DNP induced fat burning, just like exercise induced fat burning. Burning fat at an increased rate, as a result of DNP therapy or exercise, will make you sweat because it is a hot process. You get a little tired in both cases because your body is depleted of ATP. It may on rare occasion cause a headache because of dehydration.

This sentence, with its five symptoms, if taken as a whole sounds alarming. As you have just seen, the reality is that it is all smoke and mirrors when you really take a closer look at it. Now let me ask you a question: If DNP truly did harm to the body, like tobacco does, e.g. cancer, emphysema etc., would anyone ever bother to lump together these innocuous symptoms? Even if they did, they would certainly include the more serious deleterious effects. They don't here, why? The reason is because there are no such symptoms.

This smoke and mirrors sentence is both an example and proof of this book's assertion that, there is no real or solid claim of DNP harming the body. The fact is that it is impossible to find one substantial claim that is actually corroborated by a clinical study or other real life evidence. Why? It is impossible to find because DNP does not harm the body at therapeutic doses, and is only harmful if overdosed. .

Chronic oral exposure in humans and animals has resulted in formation of cataracts and skin lesions. [19]

OK, we have been over the cataracts issue. One in one thousand women who used DNP got cataracts, which means cataracts is a very rare allergic reaction that occurs in women almost exclusively.

"Skin lesions" is a bit dramatic, as this side effect is described as a rash by all the doctors and clinicians, whose work I have read. I suppose "skin lesions" is a lot scarier sounding, but this is a clinical term for "rash." This is an allergic reaction that, according to clinicians, roughly seven percent of users get. All modern day DNP users who I know of claim that over the counter antihistimes clear up this rash. Also, fifty percent of those who get the rash get over the reaction with continued use. Basically, that is a net three and one half percent allergic reaction that is easily dealt with today because of antihistamines. "Skin lesions", shish!

> *Chronic oral exposure in humans and animals has... caused effects on the bone marrow, central nervous system, and cardiovascular system.* [19]

Can someone please tell me what the heck "caused effects" means? Are they good, bad or indifferent *"effects"*? I absolutely guarantee you that if you eat a donut you will certainly *"cause effects on the bone marrow, central nervous system, and cardiovascular system"* Don't bet me on that or you will lose. What are they saying?? If they are trying to say bad "effects" then they are lying. Listen to the clinicians, there is no proof of this claim at all:

> *Dinitro treatment respects the liver, the kidneys, the cardio-vascular system and the blood. Dinitrophenol is remarkable for its absence of effect on the cardio-vascular system. Even when the basal metabolism is found elevated to significant levels, there is no change in the rhythm of the pulse (Rosenblum).* [2]

One of the most striking features of the metabolic stimulation of dinitrophenol is a lack of significant changes in blood pressure or pulse rate, unless therapeutic doses are exceeded. That is, the metabolism may be increased by as much as 50 per cent without demonstrable changes in circulatory activity. [2]

The fact is besides established by physiologists, since dinitrophenol raises thermogenesis and not the metabolic quotient. [2]

Tainter, Stockton and Cutting have reported a series of cases in which one had measured the plasma bile index and determined the test of Van de Bergh. Their analyses demonstrate, beyond a doubt, that the liver does not suffer any damage in the course of dinitro treatment.

Experimental studies on animals do not show toxic effects of dinitrophenol on the kidney (Taitner, Cutting, Wood and Proescher). Anatomical-pathological examinations of animals, even those which died from a massive dose of dinitrophenol, do not reveal any important anatomical changes, except a small degree of cytolysis. Clinical documents are not abundant, but, on the whole, do not seem to demonstrate that dinitrophenol is toxic for the kidneys.

As T.L. Schulte and M.L. Tainter wrote, "it doesn't seem that dinitrophenol at usual clinical doses is likely to harm the kidneys.

All the clinicians know actually that dinitro medication is irreplaceable in cases of monstrous obesities which prevent all exercise. It can be used in the obese for whom occupations, life style or cardiac troubles do not permit physical exercises. It is indispensible for the grossly obese in cases of abdominal operations and immobilization due to illness (inflammation of fallopian tubes, appendicitis, etc.) for which there is an urgency to obtain a reduction of subcutaneous fat.[2]

Look, no bad effects on cardiovascular system! None in the kidneys or liver! The same is said of bone marrow, in the bone marrow reference they are probably speaking of. Blood cells being affected through bone marrow are the issue there. This quote comes at the end of a rather lengthy and detailed discussion on the cardiovascular system, blood and with a reference about bone marrow. They clearly state these effects do not happen. It is in Cutting and Tainter's 1934 Stanford University Report, printed in clinical reports section of this book.

So why say it "causes effects" to the cardiovascular system? We know from clinical studies that it doesn't in any real sense implied in that quote. The same goes for the other two claims as well. If you think about it, that is why it says "caused effects". That is such vague language the writer(s) of this piece of governmental propaganda were obviously sufficiently aware of these quotes I've given that they just say "caused effects". That way, they can give the impression they want to without actually saying it. Look, I don't give a rat's rear-end about whoever wrote this and their relative culpability for their propagandist approach to governing. The bigger point here is that they are forced to go to these lengths when they discuss DNP, because they don't have any really serious side effects to discuss!

Just look at the side effects of Adderall®, one of the most prescribed drugs in the USA. Even if, for the sake of argument, everything they were claiming were true about DNP, it would be a breath mint compared to that legal drug. The list of side effects for Adderall® is shocking. The same is true of Vicodin's® list of sides and it is truly deadly, in the sense that it is easily and often overdosed. I am not saying these drugs should be banned, I am saying, that DNP should not be. You can see the side effects of these two drugs in the section, on the comparison of side effects and benefits, of several legal drugs, with those of DNP.

Ok, one paragraph down, three to go:

No information is available on adverse reproductive or developmental effects of 2,4-dinitrophenol in humans. According to available animal studies, fetal growth inhibition, but no birth defects, were reported in the offspring of animals fed 2,4-dinitrophenol. [19]

Well, it's not exactly accurate to say no information is available. After all, an estimated five hundred thousand to one million Americans used DNP over the five-year period that it was legal and most of them were women. Much of that use was clinical or prescription. Also Doctor Bachinsky prescribed it to over 14,000 patients at his clinics in the 1980's, until the FDA finally managed to shut him down.

There is no evidence of any kind that DNP did harm to any pregnancy or to women's reproductive systems from this more recent use. I would think we would have at least some inkling that it caused such adverse effects. After all, we know of two allergies that only affect a tiny fraction of users. Something like damaging fetuses or messing up reproductive works, would not be an allergic reaction. It would be dose dependant and would manifest itself prodigiously. If nothing else, there would be a history of lawsuits.

As far as, *fetal growth inhibition is concerned,* it makes sense that if you gave a mouse DNP while it was pregnant there might be a slight drop off in their offspring's weight. After all the DNP ingesting mother mice would have less energy and fat than the control mice. But there was no damage or deformity to the cute little baby mice from the DNP.

Gee, I wonder if we could extrapolate anything from those two facts. Well, it sure is amazing how the EPA can suddenly become agnostics when the known facts don't fit the party line and yet in the previous paragraph, they can imply all sorts of inaccuracies along with some outright untruths thrown in to paint their preconceived negative picture of DNP. Hmm, is it just me, or are you beginning to see a pattern here? No real reason for the ban on DNP, so make vague implications about how dangerous and damaging this "poisonous substance" is.

> *Cancer: No information is available on the carcinogenic effects of 2,4-dinitrophenol in humans. Results from one oral study in mice indicated no tumor formation occurred after six months exposure, and in another study results indicated 2,4-dinitrophenol did not promote tumor development in mice. The International Agency for Research on Cancer and the U.S. EPA have not classified 2,4-dinitrophenol for potential human carcinogenicity.* [19]

To begin with, everything I said about the previous paragraph applies here in exactly the same way.

The EPA brought up cancer, but won't even bother to point out, that all the evidence points to DNP's not being carcinogenic. They just sort of cryptically state, that it has not been classified as being carcinogenic. It just seems to me, that they don't like saying positive things about DNP. Instead, they just kind of smear it by ambiguously associating with cancer.

Let me spell it out a little more clearly, when the EPA states that there is no information on carcinogenic effects on humans what they are saying is, there have been no tests on humans, only on animals. As far as I know, scientists always test for cancer on animals instead of humans, because trying to cause cancer in humans is generally frowned upon, even for purposes of clinical analyses.

There is never any direct clinical evidence that DNP causes cancer, except extrapolation from trying desperately to give cute little mice cancer with DNP or whatever else they were testing. The only other evidence is from real world use by humans, for DNP or anything else.

There is absolutely no evidence from its vast use of DNP by the American people, when it was legal, that it is at all carcinogenic. Just like anything else, we know that DNP is non-carcinogenic, in the sense we can't make little mice cancerous with it, no matter how hard we try and people don't seem to get cancer at an increased rate when they take it. In addition, read the chapter "Don't Take My Work for It, Listen to the Experts," there are several clinical studies that show that not only does DNP not cause cancer in animal testing, it is in several ways, an anti-carcinogen.

This claim is at least an improvement from the first paragraph where all the claims are meaningless and inaccurate. Here they are guilty of economy with the truth, by not mentioning the animal studies, but just hold their nose and tell the truth about DNP in as unflattering away as they possibly can.

It can now be said that dinitrophenol is of definite value as a drug for treating obesity and perhaps some other metabolic disorders. In the hands of the medical profession, it can be used with the maximum benefit and with minimum deleterious results.[2]

The previous quote was made by the three Stanford clinicians after over a year of large scale human clinical studies and also outpatient prescription to roughly 4,500 patients out of those same clinics. It stands in stark contrast to the FDA piece below.

This FDA document is the last one analyzed in this chapter. It also serves the purpose of giving a more complete picture of one of the more interesting parts of DNP's history:

Never say "never again" is something you learn in FDA. Worthless or dangerous products have an annoying way of cropping up time after time. Even drugs thought to have been banned forever have come back from the dusty pages of history to afflict an unsuspecting public.[20]

Worthless? I don't think so. Several quotes that appear later in this document, make it clear, that DNP is not worthless. Take this one: "AMA's Council on Pharmacy and Chemistry echoed that advice. An editorial warned, 'A drug with the potency and effects of dinitrophenol is a two-edged sword with appalling possibilities for harm as well as good.'" That "A drug with the potency and effects of dinitrophenol" could have "Appalling possibilities for good" does not support the worthless charge. If you are thinking the authors of this FDA hit piece meant worthless, in the sense that it is dangerous, why do they say worthless *or* dangerous? No, they are hinting that it doesn't perform. They are making a vague smear. They could have just said dangerous. That would have been more accurate with the rest of their document's claims, because worthless in the sense of ineffective is something they disprove themselves about DNP in this article repeatedly.

Here is another example out of many in this document, where they state that DNP is definitely not ineffective: *"This is not as far-fetched as it may seem. Even in small doses dinitrophenol accelerates metabolism of the cells, increasing their consumption of oxygen. To meet the increased need for fuel, the body burns up fat. The body's temperature rises, and heat radiation increases."*

It may seem that I am belaboring a small point. No, this is an important point, for two reasons. The first reason is because it is an example of a technique used throughout this document, namely the *vague but inaccurate smear*. This method is used throughout this document to compensate for the fact that they have nothing truly serious to complain about with DNP. The other reason it is important is that the authors contradict their own implications with facts throughout this document, in the case of this smear as well as several others. I will point this all out as we proceed through this FDA propaganda piece.

> *The chemical 2,4-dinitrophenol is a case in point. Described in a chemical dictionary as "highly toxic" and a "severe explosion hazard when dry," this substance has been used in dyes, wood preservatives, weedkillers, photographic developers, explosives and, astonishingly, in weight-reducing products for human use.* [20]

How on earth can DNP be highly toxic, if the major clinical studies at Stanford University found that it only caused a skin rash but did no harm to any organ or system in the body? Also, after the first year of use by over one hundred thousand Americans, only 2 deaths were directly attributable to it, and those were due to overdose. The other uses sound scary, but really don't matter if DNP is not harmful. Alcohol has some of those same uses as well as other seemingly dangerous applications, but it is ingested orally by humans on a grand scale.

This is yet another vague assertion. This deceptive technique would be somewhat tolerable, if only occasionally used, but vague assertions are used every time DNP is criticized because there is no substantial danger with which to condemn DNP. The sole exception is when critics mention an allergic reaction. This reminds me of the question in the old commercial "where's the beef?"

Before 1938 it was legal under federal law to sell dinitrophenol (as it was commonly called) as a diet potion. At that time, drug makers were not required to prove that their products were safe before they put them on the market. Dozens of weight-reducing preparations containing dinitrophenol and other dangerous drugs were being sold. [20]

But reports were multiplying that dinitrophenol could maim and kill. It was included in the "Chamber of Horrors" exhibit prepared by FDA for hearings held by a Senate committee considering a bill that became the Federal Food, Drug, and Cosmetic Act of 1938. [20]

Again, this is an example of vague claims in the first sentence. Whenever the EPA does get specific here, the authors make claims clinically proven untrue or are referring to one or both of the known allergic reactions. "Maim and kill" can only refer to overdose, as the clinical testing and other popular legal use history proves. Again, there are no specifics.

"Chamber of Horrors" is just the kind of propagandist scare tactic language you would expect from the FDA, as it geared up for the big power grab of the Federal Food, Drug, and Cosmetic Act of 1938. How is it possible that the clinicians who studied DNP's effects on hundreds of people and prescribed it to thousands more called it "well tolerated at therapeutic doses" and defended its safety in great detail? How could what these clinicians said be true at all, in any way, if DNP really belonged in a "Chamber of Horrors?"

The reality is, even if you were to take every specific claim against DNP by the FDA, it would not belong in a Chamber of Horrors as much as Vicodin® and Adderall®. Just read the list of known side effects of those two legal FDA approved drugs. These two drugs are not even close to being the worst FDA approved drugs. If they don't belong in a "chamber of horrors" why does DNP? This over the top language is just another proof that the FDA is not in good faith. They aren't specific in their claims, but they sure are strident. These are the attributes of manipulation by deception.

I have become convinced, that the real catalyst for this power grabbing legislation was the desire of influential financial interests in the medical and weight loss industries, to ban DNP. Perhaps, it was an authority the FDA hankered for all along but the need to protect powerful interests from the financial threat that DNP posed was so urgent, that the FDA geared up and unfortunately succeeded in this effort.

As you can read in the "FDA Fun Facts" section of this book that agency has followed this pattern of hiding the truth and intimidating and silencing anyone promoting the truth in their efforts to protect the profits of the pharmaceutical companies. This pattern of corruption has been proven beyond any doubt. It has been stated time and again by the media, politicians, FDA whistle blowers, and countless doctors and even proven in federal court.

This power the FDA obtained, in order stop DNP from eradicating obesity is the primary means to the obscene pricing and profits for the medical and pharmaceutical industries. This incestuous relationship has become a chronic obstacle to Americans receiving the best available medical therapies. The FDA is a direct threat to our health and banning DNP is the single most destructive of all of their bad rulings.

You see, DNP is the first and most egregious example of FDA duplicity and deception in favor of big money medical interests and against the interests of the American people. Since DNP is the first casualty of FDA corruption and also so valuable and needed, DNP legalization is a critical place to fight the FDA.

In such a victory, we could once and for all strike at the FDA's power grabbing root action, and break the medical industry's cabal, that is destroying the health and wealth of the American people. Such a victory would simultaneously, virtually eradicate obesity and all health problems related to excess fat. Just think about that. I agree, these are bold claims, but if DNP is truly as safe and effective as the clinicians who studied it said it was then everything else I just said is a given.

Even though it was some 50 years ago that the chemical made headlines and helped toughen federal drug laws, dinitrophenol is by no means merely of historical interest. In April 1986, a Texas court issued an injunction to stop a doctor from using the deadly chemical in a weight-loss program in that state. Less than three months later, the doctor was again in court for violating that injunction. [20]

Deadly chemical huh? That is not what I found when I used DNP myself, as I am most obviously still alive to write this book. It's a lie. Think about it, there are no short-term dangers, as these very authors admit later in this essay, when they say that the clinicians did not test long enough to find any side effects. DNP must certainly not be deadly in the sense cyanide is, as cyanide didn't need clinical studies to prove it kills. In other words, DNP does not have some specific damage it does to body tissue, organs or systems. NONE HAVE EVER BEEN DISCOVERED!!!

If DNP has a long-term deadly danger, I have not heard one single specific description of this result, or read one example of someone who has suffered death from DNP use, here or anywhere else. DNP is deadly when you overdose it, but so is everything else and that is no reason to label it deadly.

Calling DNP deadly is a smear that these critics don't even believe themselves. This piece was written to make sure that the exposure to DNP, of the more than fourteen thousand Americans in Bachinsky's clinics did not bring about a movement to legalize it. This is so transparent. How do you explain the vague implications, the gross overstatements, the inaccuracies and most of all, the complete lack of a single specific side effect that explains their claim that DNP is deadly? All of the facts, as well as their literary duplicity overwhelmingly prove the writers of this FDA hit piece have an agenda other than the truth.

> *The doctor, Nicholas Bachynsky, operates a chain of "Physicians Clinics" throughout Texas and in several other states. Until last December the mainstay of his weight-loss program in Texas was dinitrophenol, which he dispensed under the trade name Mitcal. According to his advertising brochures, Russian-born Bachynsky learned of dinitrophenol in 1963 while translating Russian medical journals for the U.S. government. The Russians used it to keep soldiers warm in winter, he learned. The main side effect reported was weight loss.* [20]

Notice that the main side effect was weight loss.

> *This is not as far-fetched as it may seem. Even in small doses dinitrophenol accelerates metabolism of the cells, increasing their consumption of oxygen. To meet the increased need for fuel, the body burns up fat. The body's temperature rises, and heat radiation increases.* [20]

> *Bachynsky's advertising promised weight loss of up to 15 pounds a week under his program. Increased body heat is the only side effect mentioned. The brochure*

claimed that no deaths had been associated with Mitcal. (However, in 1984 FDA documented a suicide associated with an overdose of Mitcal by a professional weight lifter burdened with a number of emotional problems.) [20]

Wow! A suicide by overdose! This proves nothing other than DNP can be used to commit suicide. So can Vicodin® and many other drugs, in fact, they often are. So can cars, rope, and thousands of other things. Perhaps the FDA should require a warning on everything that can be used to commit suicide such as bridges, drugs, cars, buildings, etc. That is the obvious implication here. According to these critics, Dr. Bachynsky was being deceptive by not telling people that his therapeutic medicine can be used to commit suicide. Stupid statements like this are a result of the unrelenting effort to smear DNP with vague innuendo. The only weapon the authors of this essay have, aside from half truths, are outright untruths, which they indulge in quite a bit throughout this article.

The history of dinitrophenol tells a story far different from that portrayed in Bachynsky's brochure.

Before the turn of the century, European and American scientists studied the effects in laboratory animals of food dyes containing dinitrophenol and related compounds. They found the chemicals caused a rise in temperature, stimulated respiration, and hastened the onset of rigor mortis upon death. As a result, these dyes were banned in a number of countries, including the United States. [20]

Here we have one of the many examples of a half-truth in this essay. *"Rise in temperature,"* and *"stimulated respiration"* are both normal effects of increased fat burning. Clinicians describe these side effects as the same as those caused by exercise, which they are.

Clinicians never express alarm at these effects or describe them as a problem of any kind. These effects are also dose dependant. At stronger therapeutic doses, body temperature tends to go up one degree on average. The increased respiration is not generally noticeable at therapeutic levels in humans.

These mice were given fatal overdoses. You notice the authors only mention these two minor side effects on the massively overdosed little mice. That is because, in those same tests, the scientists noted that no harm was done to the organs or tissue, even with the massively fatal overdose the mice were given. Tainter and Cutting got the same results with dogs, after giving them near fatal doses, every day for six months.

The EPA, of course, does not mention this fact, the government propaganda pieces against DNP never do tell the truth about DNP. So all the critics have revealed here is that the scientists fatally overdosed some mice. They make it sound like DNP just kills animals in such a dramatic way, that the body stiffens more quickly than usual. The study that they misrepresent here actually disproves their position and proves my position, because it shows that even at fatal doses, DNP's action does not interact with the systems or tissues of the body in a destructive way.

Now that we know this, let's put it context:

They make the statement *"The history of dinitrophenol tells a story far different from that portrayed in Bachynsky's brochure."* I take this to mean, that they believed that Dr. Bachynsky was hiding DNP's real evil. Their proof for this is a scientific study that showed that fatally overdosed mice suffer no harm to their little bodies from this massive overdosing before it kills them. How does this prove their point? I guarantee that you can fatally over dose mice with any legal drug (In fact, drugs have to prove some level of toxicity to be considered effective). I am certain, that most of those drugs when overdosed to fatality do cause organ and or other systemic damage before death occurs.

This study of the fatal effects on mice doesn't prove anything other than that DNP is unusually easy on the body. This critical piece words every claim to make it sound like it proves the opposite and that DNP is super poisonous.

Again, the reason critics have to do this is because they do not have a legitimate reason to ban DNP, so they have to resort to any claim they can distort. Please, if you do not agree with this assessment, ask yourself the following questions: Is it just chance that critics never give a legitimate reason? Do these authors really have one or more such reasons, but these reasons have never been mentioned by some weird statistical anomaly? If that is so, where would they even get the knowledge of these dangers from, if they are stated nowhere else, as it is obvious they would have no personal experience with DNP if they believe it to be "deadly?"

Why are critics almost always so vague with their claims, if they actually have a legitimate claim, that DNP is cancer causing or heart tissue damaging? On the rare occasion they turn to specifics, they either mention one or both of the two rare allergic reactions. Critics are never specific with the "deadly" claim because they never bother to mention that it is an overdosing issue. If my facts are correct on these points, then my reasoning is too, and my facts are supported by clinical documents, among other proofs. My position is also supported by the fact that these government documents always, by necessity, follow the same vague and deceptive pattern of mischaracterization.

If I have been selective and omitted factual proofs or have simply not found them, then I will be proven wrong in the press. Please come forward and prove me wrong, if there is something I have missed.

I don't see how that is possible though, because the government would not have been so vague and deceptive if they would have had just one real reason. I have not missed any such facts or statements. I have researched so extensively, you would be shocked at the time I have spent on it. I am not just playing a mischaracterization game either. Look at my characterizations of their statements. I am fairly and accurately describing them every time.

> *Dinitrophenol next surfaced during World War I when French munitions workers experienced loss of appetite, nausea, vomiting, diarrhea, loss of weight, night sweats, weakness, headaches, and high fever. These symptoms improved when the workers were off the job for a few days.* [20]

> *The effects were most severe among alcoholics and those with liver and kidney problems. They developed extremely high temperatures, profuse sweating, and intense thirst. Death followed in a few hours.* [20]

This statement is utterly ridiculous. Any deaths are always due to overdosing. Whether you inhale, absorb, or eat it, DNP will not kill you, unless you take in enough to overdose it. These poor workers took in probably three or more grams in a day. If you inhaled the active ingredient in Vicodin,® it would surely kill you, if it was an amount that would be a fatal dose orally. They don't tell you this bit of history to educate but to deceive, why? I hope you can see the pattern by now.

> *A commission set up by the French Ministry of Munitions pinpointed dinitrophenol as the cause of the problem. (France was the only country using the compound in explosives.) The ministry took steps to protect its workers from dinitrophenol.* [20]

In the late 1920s, scientists started looking into possible therapeutic uses of dinitrophenol. In the July 15, 1933, issue of the Journal of the American Medical Association (JAMA), three Stanford University researchers reported that patients receiving daily oral doses of 3 to 5 milligrams of dinitrophenol per kilogram of body weight experienced steady weight reduction without demonstrable side effects. However, since their studies were short term -- no longer than three months -- the researchers warned that they could not be sure that toxic effects might not appear after longer use. They urged that "for the present, dinitrophenol be used only as an experimental therapeutic procedure in carefully selected patients under close observation by the physician. [20]

This is another half-truth. A year later when they had a much greater knowledge and understanding than they did in the report just quoted, the same clinicians released a comprehensive report that summed up their total knowledge of DNP from their own clinical studies, other clinical studies, prescription and non prescription use etc., the three clinicians in this report said: *"It can now be said that dinitrophenol is of definite value as a drug for treating obesity and perhaps some other metabolic disorders. In the hands of the medical profession, it can be used with the maximum benefit and with minimum deleterious results.*[2]

In the same report, they also said it should be obtainable with a physician's prescription because it might be used too freely. They also mention here, that there are dangers to using it indiscriminately. What the dangers are and are not, they have laid out in great detail in this same document. They came up with two: One is the danger of overdosing. They point out specifically that DNP was fatally dosed by an incredibly small percentage of users. Three total up to that point in time, but really only two that it can really be attributed to. This is after more than a year of popular use by over one hundred thousand prescription users. Then they go on to say: *"it is seen that neither of the other two cases was due to the use of the drug in the usual therapeutic doses. When one considers that some one hundred thousand patients have been treated with this exceedingly potent therapeutic agent, it is a matter of some gratification to know that fatalities have not been more numerous."[2]*

So, DNP is rarely overdosed and is statistically proven to be a less than normal threat for fatal overdosing. I am not saying that is their implication because though this quote does tend that way they are not sufficiently clear on that point. What I am saying is that with over one hundred thousand users, you have a sufficient sample to be past any real danger of statistical anomaly. That is also born out over the whole five-year period with only nine deaths.

The other side effect they found was a skin rash that could be minor or very serious, or somewhere in between. This allergic reaction disappears with half of the people that get it and does not return. In recent underground use it has become common knowledge that over the counter antihistamines solve this problem, for most everyone else.

So they took the worst quote for DNP, made at an earlier time when it was understandable that the clinicians would be cautious after so short of a testing period. But in the context of this later document it is an obsolete statement and totally disingenuous to use it, as it is not reflective of the ultimate conclusions of the three greatest of DNP experts.

There are statements the writers of this essay could have taken out of context from this report I am quoting from now, that would have better served their purpose. C'mon now, FDA propaganda guys, if you're going to all this trouble to paint a deceptive picture, you might as well do a good job of it.

There is a more in depth analyses of this document in the chapter on the clinical reports, at the end of the report itself. I deal with a few statements, that if taken out of context would seem to at least somewhat undermine my position, but upon closer inspection actually ultimately support it.

> *In the same issue of the journal, AMA's Council on Pharmacy and Chemistry echoed that advice. An editorial warned, "A drug with the potency and effects of dinitrophenol is a two-edged sword with appalling possibilities for harm as well as good.* [20]

> *This warning was soon borne out. In the Sept. 30, 1933, issue of JAMA, three San Francisco physicians described a severe skin reaction in a woman who had taken dinitrophenol for 14 days. They concluded the chemical was not as safe for weight reduction as other methods in common use. Then San Francisco newspapers reported the bizarre death of a Viennese doctor who took an overdose of dinitrophenol to achieve quick weight loss and, as one newspaper put it, "literally cooked to death." His temperature had reached 110 degrees Fahrenheit.* [20]

Now these essayists are really reaching. Mind you, these quotes and stories are supposed to be supporting their contention that DNP is useless and dangerous. So far, they have not managed anything that stands up to even a little scrutiny. These two events discussed in this paragraph do not either and really don't require anything more than basic common sense to understand.

This skin reaction is the first real side effect they have discussed. However, it does not support the FDA's position that DNP is dangerous and should be banned. The rash is a relatively low occurrence allergic reaction. Approximately one half of the people who develop it, quickly acquire a tolerance to DNP and no longer have the reaction. Skin rashes are one of the most common allergic reactions people have to other drugs. There are not many, perhaps any, substances that there are no people that have an allergic skin reaction to.

An allergic skin reaction is not a reason to ban a valuable drug. Those people who are not allergic can still benefit. The few who are allergic don't take it. This is the normal protocol for allergic reactions. Antibiotics have a much higher rate of allergic reaction. So why are they even bringing it up? Because they have not even one side effect serious enough to support their ban on it. If they did have one, they have ignored it in favor of half-truths, misstatements and allergies. That pattern is a fact in this document and it repeats itself in every official government proclamation of the dangers of DNP that I have read.

I will give the essayists this much: They are two for two in being accurate in this paragraph. They didn't just say he died while not mentioning it was from overdose. That is what is usually found in anti-DNP FDA propaganda. These authors have already done it more than once in this article.

The problem is it does not support their contention that DNP is dangerous. Overdosing DNP is dangerous, but overdosing anything is dangerous by definition, as if it were not dangerous, it would still be considered a safe dose. DNP is relatively harmless if not overdosed. When I say relatively, I mean even more harmless than Tylenol®. Tylenol® is hard on some organs of the body, like the liver, DNP isn't. You can overdose both. There are people allergic to both. But DNP is innocuous to the body when compared even to Tylenol®.

By the way, this guy took five grams of DNP at once. That is more than eighty times the minimum effective therapeutic dose. Imagine if a person took eighty Vicodin® or eighty Adderall® or even eighty Aspirin for that matter. That would be the last stupid thing they ever did, but it would not be proof that those drugs are so dangerous that they should be banned.

I realize most readers have not researched all of the FDA and other official statements themselves and so for the moment, only have these present examples to analyze. Just for the sake of argument, presume the claim of mine to be true, that the other quotes follow this same duplicitous pattern. Is there any other rational explanation for this behavior, than that the FDA is protecting the profits of the same industries that it has always served to protect in this fashion? There isn't. Go ahead and do your own research and you will see the same pattern repeated. Common sense tells you that the examples of FDA propaganda you have already seen make it a virtual certainty, that is exactly what you will find.

> *In a report on this death, JAMA predicted, "It is to be expected that, with the craze that has in the past few years affected the American public, and especially the feminine contingent thereof, for shortcuts to the sylph figure, proprietary products will begin to appear having for their essential drug dinitrophenol.* [20]

> *During the next 15 months an estimated 100,000 persons took the drug for weight reduction. More than 1,200,000 capsules were dispensed from a single clinic in San Francisco. More than 20 drug houses supplied both dinitrophenol and mixtures containing the drug. Proprietary products with such names as Nox-Ben-ol, Nitroment, Nitraphen, Redusols, Formula 17, Slim, Dinitrenal and Dinitrole were freely sold in drugstores without a prescription and with no warnings or adequate directions for use. Only in New Jersey, Louisiana and California was a prescription required.* [20]

It was assumed that the chief danger from this drug lay in the careless use of over-the-counter products. But physicians were reporting serious toxic reactions, including severe skin rashes, agranulocytosis (a potentially fatal blood disorder), jaundice, and disturbances of smell and taste even in patients under their care. Some deaths also were reported. Unfortunately, there was no way to predict who might suffer these reactions. [20]

Here we go again. This paragraph has it all: half-truths, untruths and allergies.

The skin rashes that are caused by DNP can be severe but they generally are not, and they only affect a small percentage of people. Agranulocytosis is not caused by DNP. This fact is discussed in great detail in the same report I have quoted from several times in analysis of this document. The three clinicians describe it by name and symptoms. They point out that because one person on DNP had this condition it was feared that the DNP may have caused it. They go into great detail explaining how they tested for this and their conclusion is that this rare blood disorder is not caused by DNP. They do say that if the person was prone to this disorder, it is theoretically possible that some substances could perhaps somehow speed up its onset and DNP could possibly be among those substances. This is simply stated as a possibility that could not be ruled out for certain, but not for any specific causative reason.

The three clinicians also address jaundice claims against DNP in the same report. They say that DNP does not cause jaundice, but that it was mistakenly thought to, because DNP can cause a yellow tint to body tissues due to the fact that it is a yellow dye. So it does not cause jaundice for sure and we know that from clinical study as well as the fact that it is not a problem that arose with the popular use.

The disturbance of smell and taste is a rare claim. It is at worst an allergic reaction, and is more probably an effect of toxins exiting the body with the excess fat. It definitely is not a serious side effect either.

Risk of death is brought up again in an extremely deceptive manner here. First, we know exactly which deaths they are referring to here as they are covered in detail in the same report I have been quoting from. They got their other facts quoted in the previous paragraph from the same report. They have put this quote specifically in the context of the first year of use because that is the time period the report covers from which they are quoting. As I mentioned earlier in this chapter, there were three deaths, two of which could be attributed to DNP overdose. One of the two was the guy they just mentioned a few paragraphs back. Yep, the "massive-5-gram-overdose-eighty-times-the-minimum-dose-guy."

They give the impression that they are piling up deaths here but they are talking about the same one multiple places. These two deaths are covered in detail by the three Stanford Clinicians who I quote in detail. They were both due to overdose. Here is another example where these essayists knew specifically that the deaths they keep referring to were caused by overdose, because it is covered in the source document they are quoting. DNP has never anywhere been specifically accused of being fatal except by overdose. It is always a deception to say "deaths" as though DNP just spontaneously kills people. The whole FDA sham is pretty much propped up on this one deception. But here we have them red handed referring to deaths they knew were caused by overdose and they deceptively hide this fact to confuse.

As I have stated several times in this book, they make the deaths claim, add on an allergic reaction or two and then sometimes add some untrue accusations. The whole sordid technique is laid out in a nice little one-paragraph package for your edification.

This FDA propaganda document is not only ineffective in accomplishing its goal, it is also a deception. It is meant to keep people ignorant of the safety and efficacy of the most valuable of all known medicine's to protect the profits of the medical industry, the survival of an obsolete weight loss industry and most of all the obscene profits of the pharmaceutical companies.

If anyone doesn't see this now, after reading the whole first half of this book and the pattern of deception repeating itself in such a sickeningly predictable manner, I have really nothing to say except that they probably deserve what the FDA is doing to them. For everyone else, please don't just let this go. It is too grave an injustice to just lie down and ignore! DNP is desperately needed by scores of millions of people in this country.

> *In August 1934, the Food and Drug Administration issued the first of a series of warnings, pointing out that sales of dinitrophenol fat reducers were booming, despite the reports of deaths, but the 1906 Food and Drugs Act did not cover products of this type. All FDA could do was to warn the public.* [20]

> *Nevertheless, the agency was preparing for action -- to test the law if nothing else. Chemists at FDA's Chicago district laboratory were involved in a crash project analyzing a broad range of reducing products. Dinitrophenol was found in products that did not reveal their contents on the label. An official method of analysis for dinitrophenol was developed and sent out to cooperating enforcement agencies in the states.* [20]

Notice that after only one year of use the FDA was already after DNP. This is at the same time the definitive report on DNP was released. This is a very important fact that proves something I suspected, but had only found one other proof until I found it in this document. I go into greater detail about this in my analyses of that report in this book. Thanks FDA propaganda guys for proving what I suspected to be true.

> *At the same time, the E. I. DuPont de Nemours Company informed FDA that it was trying to restrict its sales of dinitrophenol to industrial users.* [20]

I wonder how much DuPont's other business was suffering from the very inexpensive DNP wiping out all other weight loss drugs and pharmaceutical sales?

> *In April 1935, a virtual epidemic of cataracts began to occur, predominantly in young women who had been taking dinitrophenol. Some cases showed up months or years after the last dose of the drug had been taken. Tragically, once started, changes in the eye's lens progressed rapidly until vision was obscured. Dr. Warren D. Homer, a San Francisco ophthalmologist and one of the first to report dinitrophenol-related cataracts, estimated that more than 164 people were affected. Newspaper headlines proclaimed "Blinded By Drug To Reduce Weight," "Anti-Fat Drug May Cause Blindness," and "Women Blinded In Reducing Try." [20]*

This is the official reason that the FDA gave for banning DNP for fat reduction therapy. While I have already covered this somewhat, I need to clear up some inaccuracies in the above paragraph. The authors state that there was an 'epidemic" of cataracts. It was not an epidemic in the sense that a lot of people were affected, or even a high ratio of people. It is because 164 out of 177 cases happened in an 18-month period. That proves beyond any real doubt that the culprit was some impurity in the supply of one company or some other anomaly. (Also, there is reason to believe most of those 164 cases happened in California.)

Let's do a little math to give the overall ratio of occurrence to show that it was no epidemic, in the true sense of the word. There were a reported 177 cases of cataracts in 500,000 users over five years. That is roughly one in every 3,000 DNP users. The FDA conveniently rounds this up to one percent in their estimates. That's fine considering it's all they had, aside from the rare overdosing and they could not use that without really looking stupid.

In the "Three Real Health Concerns" chapter I go into a lot more detail on this issue.

On July 6, 1935, the AMA's Council on Pharmacy and Chemistry reported dinitrophenol would not be included in its quasi-official list of acceptable remedies. [20]

In September 1935, FDA Commissioner Walter Campbell repeated the previous year's warning against dinitrophenol, this time stressing the danger of blindness: "The eye cataracts develop with a rapidity and malignancy hitherto unknown, and result in total blindness within a comparatively short time." [20]

Campbell pointed out that existing federal law was "silent with respect to the control of dangerous drugs," and that the only possible application of the law would be through "some misstatement of fact or fraudulent curative claim in the labeling." In any event, he said, "the law can be invoked only when the product has been transported across a State line." He said the agency, contrary to its usual policy, "would take advantage of any legal technicality in proceeding against all products containing dinitrophenol." [20]

Such technicalities were found in two cases against a product called "Slim." The reducing pills were labeled as "safe to use," whereas medical opinion was unanimous to the contrary. Three shipments were seized -- two in Pittsburgh and one in Fort Wayne, Ind. The seizures were not contested in court and the products were destroyed. [20]

Though dinitrophenol made headlines in the papers and news reports on radio, it took another experience to demonstrate effectively the need for a stronger drug law -- the 107 deaths in 1937 from a poisonous elixir of sulfanilamide. In this disaster, a popular sulfa drug had been dissolved in diethylene glycol, a deadly poison. The chemist tested the solvent for flavor, appearance and fragrance but, unfortunately, not for safety. [20]

The only remedy for such a situation, said FDA Commissioner Campbell, was a law "which will require that all medicines placed upon the market shall be safe for use under the directions for use, and for potent drugs and new drugs a federal licensing system is probably the answer." [20]

In 1938, the Federal Food, Drug, and Cosmetic Act was enacted, giving FDA the power to take action against drugs that are dangerous even when used in the recommended dosage. Subsequently, the agency included dinitrophenol in a list of drugs potentially so toxic that they should not be used even under a physician's supervision. [20]

Apparently manufacturers had already gotten the message. Reducing potions containing dinitrophenol disappeared from the marketplace. FDA's Annual

Report for 1940 was able to state: "Again, as in 1939, no articles containing dinitrophenol were encountered." [20]

Since that time no drug containing this dangerous chemical has been approved by FDA for any use in humans. [20]

Again "dangerous" is thrown around loosely. Vague repetition of the same smears over and over. I won't even bother to point out all of them.

Dinitrophenol's notorious history was not unknown to Dr. Bachynsky; he cited the medical reports of the 1930s in a paper he hoped to publish and which he made available to FDA. But that did not stop him from using the chemical in his weight-loss clinics. In fact, his brochure stated that his was the only program in the nation using this substance. In addition, he claims to have discovered that dinitrophenol "decreases useful energy production, and thus makes an over-efficient metabolism very inefficient," so subjects can burn off unwanted fat. Treatment at Bachynsky's clinics was not cheap -- in the neighborhood of $1,300. [20]

Although Bachynsky's brochure stated, "There have been no fatalities associated with Mitcal," the consent form patients were asked to sign lists among the potential risks of his treatment "blood clots in veins and lungs; cataract formation; hemorrhage; allergic reactions; and even death." This apparently wasn't enough to dissuade prospective patients. As many as 14,000 people were treated at Bachynsky's clinics, according to court papers. [20]

FDA first learned of the clinics in late 1982 when some of Bachynsky's customers started calling the agency's Houston office to complain of adverse reactions, including fever, shortness of breath, dizziness and sweating. [20]

The last two paragraphs totally prove my position that DNP's side effects are the exactly the same as the side effects that result from exercise and only those. 14,000 people were given DNP therapy in the 1980's and the list of reported *"adverse reactions"* includes *"fever, shortness of breath, dizziness and sweating" That's* it! Where is the death, the toxicity, the danger or the poisonous action on the body? The FDA propagandists who wrote this document would have never included this list if they knew my book would be written, because my book makes this point constantly. Whether they caught this inconsistency or not, they felt safe to include it. Looks like I caught you FDA propaganda guys red handed again. The truth comes out! Those symptoms are the same side effects that result from exercise. These symptoms are all that was recorded after 14,000 people used DNP and these FDA Bozos admitted it.

FDA investigators went to Bachynsky's Houston clinic and to the pharmacy next door, also owned by Bachynsky, where they observed bulk containers of dinitrophenol from the Eastman Kodak Co. labeled "For chemical purposes, not for drug use." The pharmacy appeared to be using this material to compound Mitcal. The FDA investigators warned Bachynsky that he was using a dangerous, unapproved drug in violation of federal law. [20]

In March 1983 Bachynsky wrote to FDA's Houston office that since Mitcal was not for sale, distribution or transportation across state lines, the clinic was not breaking any laws. Mitcal was not sold to patients at the clinic or anywhere else; it was part of the total treatment. Since the raw material in Mitcal had been shipped across state lines, FDA did have jurisdiction but, in the agency's opinion, a case against Bachynsky for use of an unapproved new drug was better handled by the state; federal law does not regulate the practice of medicine. [20]

In 1985 Bachynsky opened a new clinic in Dallas. Soon complaints of adverse reactions to his treatment began to come in to the agency's Dallas office and to a local poison control center. FDA wrote to Bachynsky on Aug. 19, 1985, pointing out again that dinitrophenol is a "new drug" needing FDA approval. In addition, the letter explained that under the Texas Food, Drug, and Comestic Act new drugs cannot be sold, or even given away, unless they have been approved by FDA or have been tested and found safe, and an application for marketing has been filed with the Texas commissioner of health. This had not been done, according to the commissioner. [20]

Such approval was not necessary, Bachynsky responded, since the Texas law does not apply to a drug sold in the state before the enactment of the 1938 Federal Food, Drug, and Cosmetic Act. In support of his claim that dinitrophenol is safe for weight control, he enclosed his paper describing clinical trials with the drug. Furthermore, he said a "pre-IND" submission had already been sent to FDA headquarters. (An IND is a request for an exemption to federal drug laws and is filed to permit testing of an investigational new drug on humans. Bachynsky's submission was, in effect, a "testing of the waters.") [20]

Texas authorities were not convinced by Bachynsky's response to FDA that his use of dinitrophenol was legal. In November 1985, the Texas attorney general brought suit against the doctor and his clinics. The state charged that, among other things, Bachynsky failed to advise his patients that the drug is not generally recognized as safe for weight loss, that it is highly toxic, and that it is not approved by FDA. [20]

Supporting the state's case were a written affidavit and a videotaped deposition by Dr. Robert Temple, director of the Office of Drug Research and Review in FDA's Center for Drugs and Biologics. In both, Dr. Temple discussed the toxicity and the adverse effects of dinitrophenol. He pointed out that although it was widely used in the 1930s, there have been no published reports of adequate, well-controlled clinical studies showing that the drug is safe. [20]

What exactly are the toxic effects? I still have not seen any. It is no smear, but an outright lie to say that there were no adequate published reports. The Stanford clinical studies report I have quoted from throughout this book, meet or exceed any standard for controlled clinical studies. The only problem Dr. Robert Temple of the FDA has with this report and the over one year of clinical studies at one of the most prestigious university clinics in the country is that it's conclusions don't agree with the lies he is telling here so he just dismisses it all as not acceptable. The FDA is an obstacle to American health and has been for a long time.

The case against Bachynsky came to trial on March 10, 1986, in Dallas. On March 21 the jury found him guilty of drug law violations and ordered him to pay $86,000 in fines and attorney's fees. The presiding judge, Leonard Hoffman, immediately issued an injunction *prohibiting Bachynsky from dispensing dinitrophenol to any patients. The final judgment, handed down on April 10, provides that the defendants may use dinitrophenol only if it is approved by FDA or if FDA allows its use under an IND. [20]*

Bachynsky apparently was not deterred by the orders of the court any more than he was by the history of dinitrophenol. In July, the doctor and his Dallas clinic were charged with violating the April injunction by continuing to solicit patients with the intent of dispensing dinitrophenol, by representing that the drug is safe for use in a weight-loss program, and by failing to advise patients that the drug is a highly toxic herbicide (weedkiller). [20]

DNP may be an herbicide but it is not highly toxic at low doses. These critics lump a vague unsubstantiated claim together with a dangerous sounding, but actually harmless to humans industrial use of DNP.

Because of the large amount of money Bachynsky made from his Texas customers (in excess of $8 million), the court decided the penalty would not be meaningful unless it was substantial. Therefore, Bachynsky and the clinic were fined a total of $100,000, with interest at the rate of 10 percent a year beginning Aug. 1, 1986, the day the judgment was signed. [20]

Bachynsky continues to operate the Physicians Clinics, though he is now using substances other than dinitrophenol for weight reduction. The clinic program has been expanded to include treatments for impotence and smoking cessation. Dinitrophenol has not been abandoned completely, however. Bachynsky presented the results of his studies with the chemical to an FDA advisory committee in September 1986. He said he hoped that the committee would have an open mind if he submits an IND in the future. [20]

Committee members felt that if the question of whether dinitrophenol is an effective treatment for obesity is reopened, it should be done in the classic fashion with rigorous testing of the drug in animals first and then with very carefully monitored studies in people under hospital conditions. [20]

So whatever happened to those clinical studies? They never happened and they never will, as long as the pharmaceutical companies-eerrr- FDA has its way.

This article was published in the February 1987 issue of FDA Consumer. At the time it was written, Ms. Hecht was a member of FDA's public affairs staff and Mr. Janssen is FDA's historian. In 1990, Bachynsky's Texas medical license was canceled after he was sentenced to prison in a case involving insurance fraud. [20]

I wonder what caused the government to go after this doctor for insurance fraud? I'm just asking.

It should be noted here, that with over 14,000 people treated, there were no deaths, no records of long-term injury or harm and no lawsuits from the patients. If DNP were truly dangerous or harmful this would be impossible.

Figure 3

2,4-Dinitrophenol is a potent uncoupler of oxidative phosphorylation, and may cause methemoglobinemia. [20]

Wrong again FDA guys. The quote below is a classic description of methemoglobinemia and it is shown by these clinical doctors not to occur with therapeutic DNP treatment.

In studying the possibility that dinitrophenol might affect the blood, both the red and white corpuscles must be considered. Thus far we have not made extensive red cell counts in patients receiving dinitrophenol, but there have been no evidences of anemia, even after months of medication. The oxygen capacity of the blood of 15 patients was determined for possible evidences of injury to the respiratory function of the blood. Since the normal oxygen capacity of the blood varies from 18 to 21 vols. per cent and in these medicated patients the average value was 19.5 vols. per cent with a range of from 18 to 22 per cent, there is no reason to believe that the blood was injured. These patients received an average of 0.3 gm. sodium dinitrophenol daily, for an average period of 6 weeks. The addition of sodium dinitrophenol, in concentrated solution to several specimens of blood did not change the oxygen capacity. Therefore, the drug does not appear to affect the hemoglobin of the blood in vitro and in vivo.[2]

Study was also made of the fragility of the red cells of these same patients to determine whether there was any increased tendency of the cells to hemolyze. The cells were exposed to various strengths of hypotonic salt solution and the concentrations at which hemolysis began and was complete were noted.29 Hemolysis of normal cells begins at from 0.46 to 0.38 per cent concentration and is complete at from 0.34 to 0.25 per cent. With the cells of the medicated patients, the hemolysis began at an average of 0.44 per cent, with a range of from 0.42 to 0.46 percent, and was complete at an average of 0.31 per cent, with a range from 0.25 to 0.38 per cent. Since these values were all within the normal range, there was no evidence of alteration in fragility of the red cells.[2]

CHAPTER TEN

FDA Fun Facts

This books assertion that the FDA is acting wrongly regarding its continued ban on DNP, is based on a line of reasoning that has a logical sequence:

1. First, the fact that DNP is both safe and effective, when used properly, according to every fact and measure in the public record. Sure, there is a lot of negative opinion of DNP, but is never expressed by anyone that has had direct experience with it. It is mostly just people parroting what they've read of FDA originated propaganda. Whether doctors or patients in the past or modern day underground users today, if they attack DNP it is because they only know what they've been propagandized to believe. The opposite is the case with those that have personal experience with DNP. They always speak of its effectiveness and never claim they have been harmed by it in any way.

2. Since DNP is capable of burning off ten to fifteen pounds of fat a month, and can do it safely, it would make all other known fat loss chemicals and therapies obsolete. It would also mean that people would become much healthier on average in this country. All of this is good for the people that need DNP, but is a huge economic threat to people in the weight loss and medical industries. These first two logical steps lead to the FDA, because it has been the attack dog on the DNP front all along. Now there is a third fact that makes this all the more believable. The FDA has a pattern of serving the interests of these industries, especially in the pharmaceutical sector. If you really take a hard look at the incestuous relationship between the pharmaceutical industry and the FDA, you can see that the Pharmaceutical companies have a monopoly that is a direct

consequence of the FDA's entire mode of operation. Whether you believe that the FDA is corrupt or not, it cannot be denied that the pharmaceutical industry is, on a dollar for dollar basis, the most profitable industry because of the monopoly it possesses as a direct result of the FDA. It is a practical reality that supplying and maintaining this monopoly is the primary function of the FDA.

3. So, the third and final step in the logical sequence is that the FDA is both the guardian and provider of the big pharmaceutical industries extremely profitable monopoly. I have said enough in this book about how government is often corrupted in favor of special interests. The statements in this chapter from a variety of sources show how the FDA is corrupt in this sense to its very core.

There is no need for me to comment further on the statements in this chapter. They speak for speak for themselves. Note: All of the following statements are direct quotes from sources listed:

- The FDA has been in the line of fire for serious violations of its mission. The charge: Standing up for pharmaceutical profits, rather than the health of those people who are using medicines.[21]
- Under the FDA's rule, pharmaceutical companies have become the most profitable industry on planet earth, but our health is not getting any better - rather the reverse. Every year, national budgets are straining to meet increasing costs of healthcare, much of which goes to expensive, but evidently quite useless pharmaceuticals.[21]
- The companies that produce patentable medicines have the FDA in their pockets. They control the agency that is supposed to oversee their operations. The tool: user fees, which pay much of the FDA's budget, but which come with strings attached. The money may be used to expedite the approval of

new pharmaceutical drugs, but not to monitor their safety once they are on the market. [21]

- In 1992, Congress authorized the FDA to collect funds directly from the drug manufacturers. [22]

- The fact that the FDA is dependent on drug industry money is, at minimum, a conflict of interest and more likely, financial dependence on the drug manufacturers represents the corruption of a public agency. The FDA receiving funding from the organizations that they are mandated to monitor, is similar to the FBI receiving funding from the mafia. [22]

- I have been a senior healthcare executive for more than 20 years. When I first started my thesis research I had no idea that the FDA was receiving a significant portion of its funding from the drug industry. At the time I started the study, even if I had known of the FDA's financial relationship to the drug industry, I wouldn't have believed that the FDA could be corrupted or influenced by this funding method. After two-years of investigation, I am convinced that the FDA's dependence on drug industry fees has created a deadly, unethical alliance and caused a principal-agent, pro-drug industry shift, that puts millions of innocent Americans at risk. In my opinion, due to its dependence on drug industry fees, the FDA's actions related to prescription drugs are suspect, and the Agency can no longer be trusted to act in its traditional capacity as a legitimate, objective, consumer protection agency[22]

- User fees may, in fact, be creating new problems. Large businesses can readily afford the substantial fees for filing applications with FDA, but to smaller firms, these fees are a sizeable burden. Consider, for example, that user fees can cost a sponsor of a new drug over $500,000 for a single application, and the fees associated with new medical devices and biologics can exceed $150,000.[22]

- The departure of the Food and Drug Administration's chief David Kessler will close a chapter on one of the country's worst regulatory regimes. The question now is whether the abuses that characterized his regime will set a pattern for future regulators or whether they will be a lesson on the deadly consequences of placing unchecked power in the hands of unelected bureaucrats.[23]
- Federal law requires the FDA to evaluate the safety and efficacy of pharmaceuticals and medical devices. The actual testing is done by manufacturers and private laboratories, not the FDA. That agency is not an Underwriters Laboratories; it is an agency of paper shufflers. Today, by a conservative estimate, on average it takes eight years and costs nearly $400 million to bring a new medicine to market. Much of that time is spent administering FDA-mandated tests, not for safety but efficacy, and complying with other FDA requirements. During those delays thousands of Americans die and countless others suffer needlessly[23]
- Kessler himself actually defined the fundamental problem with the FDA when he spoke concerning the choice to use breast implants, "It has become fashionable in some quarters to argue that women ought to be able to make such decisions on their own. If members of our society were empowered to make their own decisions about the entire range of products for which the FDA has responsibility, however, then the whole rationale for the agency would cease to exist." Quite so! And that is the issue that Congress should consider as it determines the future of the FDA.[23]

From: "FDA Suffers Second Massive Legal Defeat in "Pearson vs. Shalala II"

The Court ruled the FDA's health claim standard to be arbitrary and capricious because it was so subjective that no one could determine precisely what level of scientific evidence FDA expected in order to approve a claim. It ordered FDA to define a new standard comprehensibly—something that FDA has still not done. It told FDA that even in the presence of a defined standard the agency would be expected to allow health claims except in the narrowest of circumstances: when it proved with empirical evidence that a health claim was not only misleading to consumers but also that it could not be rendered nonmisleading through the addition of a disclaimer. Pearson I made disclosure over suppression the order of the day. FDA was supposed to implement the decision immediately, fully and faithfully. FDA did not. In fact, FDA still has not done so.[24]

The current emphasis is on freedom of truthful information. The **Health Freedom Protection Act (H.R. 2117)** was introduced by Congressman Ron Paul in the House of Representative on May 2, 2007. Congressman Paul is a staunch believer in our constitutional rights. It is also interesting to keep in mind that Congressman Paul is a physician who is very concerned about our health. Congressman Paul asked Attorney Emord to write the Congressional bill. In the introduction to the bill, Congressman Paul states in part:

> *"This bill restores the First Amendment rights of consumers to receive truthful information regarding the benefits of foods and dietary supplements by codifying the First Amendment standards used by Federal courts to strike down the Food and Drug Administration (FDA) efforts to censor truthful health claims. The Health Freedom Protection Act also stops the Federal Trade Commission (FTC) from censoring truthful*

health care claims. The American people have made it clear they do not want the Federal government to interfere with their access to dietary supplements, yet the FDA and the FTC continue to engage in heavy-handed attempts to restrict such access. The FDA continues to frustrate consumers' efforts to learn how they can improve their health even after Congress, responding to a record number of constituents' comments, passed the Dietary Supplement and Health and Education Act of 1994 (DSHEA). FDA bureaucrats are so determined to frustrate consumers' access to truthful information that they are even evading their duty to comply with four Federal court decisions vindicating consumers' First Amendment rights to discover the health benefits of foods and dietary supplements. FDA bureaucrats have even refused to abide by the DSHEA section allowing the public to have access to scientific articles and publications regarding the role of nutrients in protecting against diseases by claiming that every article concerning this topic is evidence of intent to sell a drug. Because of the FDA's censorship of truthful health claims, millions of Americans may suffer with diseases and other health care problems they may have avoided by using dietary supplements. For example, the FDA prohibited consumers from learning how folic acid reduces the risk of neural tube defects for 4 years after the Centers for Disease Control and Prevention recommended every woman of childbearing age take folic acid supplements to reduce neural tube defects. This FDA action contributed to an estimated 10,000 cases of preventable neutral tube defects! The FDA also continues to prohibit consumers from learning about the scientific evidence that glucosamine and chondroitin sulfate are effective in the treatment of osteoarthritis; that omega-3 fatty acids may reduce the risk of sudden death heart attack; and that calcium may reduce the risk of bone fractures. The Health Freedom Protection Act will force the FDA to at last comply with the commands of Congress, the First Amendment, and the American people by codifying the First Amendment standards adopted by the Federal courts. Specifically, the Health Freedom Protection Act stops the FDA from censoring truthful claims about the curative, mitigative, or preventative effects of dietary supplements, and adopts the Federal court's suggested use of disclaimers as an alternative to censorship. The Health Freedom Protection Act also stops the FDA from prohibiting the distribution of scientific articles and publications regarding the role of nutrients in protecting against disease. This legislation also addresses the FTC's violations of the First Amendment. Under traditional First Amendment jurisprudence, the Federal government bears the burden of proving an advertising statement false before censoring that statement. However, the FTC has reversed the standard in the case of dietary supplements by requiring supplement manufactures to satisfy an unobtainable standard of proof that their statement is true. The FTC's standards are blocking innovation in the marketplace."[25]

In a June 2007 news article for Apostille.us, Stephen Fox said, "Senate Bill S.1082 and House bill HR.1561 could result in sweeping FDA "reform." Will this legislation accomplish anything beneficial? Lobbyists from Big Pharma were able to influence the Senate to neutralize any real reform. Buried within this legislation is an attack on dietary supplements. The FDA has always challenged dietary supplements because they are safer and more effective than drugs. FDA acts as a police-force bully to crush competition and keep Americans ignorant about proven homeopathic venues to treat and to prevent illnesses. Bill S.1082 permits FDA to apply drug-related risk benefit analysis to the safety of food and dietary supplements and remove commonly used products from the market at their whim."[26, 27]

CHAPTER ELEVEN

Line of Reasoning
(In a Nutshell)

The very essence of this work's theses boils down to this: that DNP does not have a single specific claim against it that justifies the FDA banning it from use as a prescription medicine. Not in the clinical studies performed on it, and not in the record of its widespread medical use by hundreds of thousands of Americans when it was legal.

There is an abundance of innuendo, name-calling, warnings etc. but none of this is based on the extensive clinical testing or the vast experience with it as a prescription medicine. For example, if there was a

> **FACT: Obesity increases the risk of Sleep apnea and respiratory problems.**
> http://www.cdc.gov/nccdphp/dnpa/obesit

clinical study or a pattern arising from the experience of real world prescription and non-prescription use, that DNP causes damage to the kidneys or cardiovascular system or endocrine system etc. But there is no such study, and no such pattern. If DNP were shown to bring on some chronic condition in a sufficient percentage of users to be categorized more than an allergic reaction. But there is no evidence of this either. No one makes either of these claims against DNP, at least not specifically and definitively.

There are only two specific claims of DNP's danger that are not strictly related to overdosing. The first is that less than 1% of women who used it got cataracts. The second is that roughly 7% of all patients got a rash. These two symptoms are analyzed in more detail as to their import and veracity in other parts of this book.

The cataract issue is the official reason that the FDA banned DNP. Even if one tenth of one percent of users developed cataracts, that effect would be at worst an allergic reaction. No valuable medicine is pulled from public use because such a small percentage of people have such a relatively rare and usually curable side effect. But that is exactly what the FDA did. Remember, DNP burns fat off at with amazing efficiency. So well, in fact, that it would be hard to improve on it. DNP is not harmful and it is the perfect solution to the biggest health issue facing mankind. It should be treated like every other medicine. People who are discovered to be allergic, either get treated for their allergic reaction or simply don't take it.

There are a great many FDA sanctioned prescription medicines that have far inferior benefits and far worse side effects, both more serious and frequent. See the section comparing DNP to other medications and therapies for specifics.

To keep this all in context, it is important to remember that DNP use by prescription alone was over 100,000 Americans in just the first year after the first clinical studies were released, in 1933. A conservative estimate of DNP users for the five years it was a legally prescribed substance, range from 500,000 to 1,000,000 Americans. This amount of use is certainly sufficient to discover any dangerous side effects that DNP might cause. If there were some specific deleterious effect on the body, it would have manifested itself as a pattern and been commented on somewhere. More likely, a lot of discussion would have ensued in the medical community or popular media and most of all by the FDA when it was banned.

The following list will serve as a distinct line of reasoning that encompasses the rationale of this book. It is a logical sequence outlining the assertions that are analyzed and proven with facts and reason throughout this book. It should be understood that three exceptions apply to many of the individual assertions. These are: (1)That DNP can be dangerous or fatal if overdosed (like everything else you can put in your mouth) (2)That under one tenth of one percent

118

of DNP users may have gotten cataracts. (3)That seven percent of DNP users develop a rash.

The line of reasoning.

- ✓ DNP was at one time a legally prescribed medical therapy for fat reduction in the United States.

- ✓ It was fabulously successful and incredibly effective as a prescription medicine for fat reduction.

- ✓ It was clinically proven to burn fat at an incredible and unprecedented rate.

- ✓ At clinical therapeutic doses it is more effective at fat reduction than any other substance by a huge factor.

- ✓ Its effective action, biochemically speaking, is equivalent to exercise and has virtually no risks or side effects that exercise doesn't have. (This assertion is made by top clinical experts after extensive large scale clinical testing at some of the world's most prestigious clinics.)

- ✓ It's mode of action on basal metabolism fat burning is so simple and effective it would be difficult to imagine a specific realistic improvement to it.

- ✓ After 5 years of legal prescription and non-prescription use by hundreds of thousands of Americans, DNP was banned by the FDA in 1938 for causing cataracts in one in one thousand users (almost exclusively women). This bizarre decision flew in the face of the position of most of the eminent clinicians and their studies, that clearly asserted DNP to be "well tolerated at therapeutic doses", extremely effective and indispensable.

✓ The cataract side effect affecting one in one thousand women is at worst, a rarely occurring allergic reaction and certainly no justification for the FDA to ban such a valuable medical therapy, by any rational standard.

✓ The fact that the FDA mentions this as the sole reason, is a pitiful proof that there is no seriously harmful side effect. They would surely have included such a reason in their banning proclamation. It also forces the question as to what special interests were served by such an inexplicable and numbingly costly decision for the American people.

✓ There are catastrophic financial ramifications for two large and powerful industries if DNP was returned to legal prescription drug status. In at least a passive sense, this is the only motive and the intuitively obvious factor behind the FDA's failure to reverse the tragic decision to ban DNP.

✓ Additionally, the FDA has been proven beyond any doubt to act on the behalf of the profits of the pharmaceutical industry.

✓ From the ban until the present, in the FDA statements, medical journals and all other reports with any kind of official medical authority behind them, there is no specific claim of long-term injury of any kind to the body.

✓ It was extensively clinically tested and found to not be harmful to the human body eg. (DNP does no known damage to the heart or cardiovascular system, kidneys, liver etc

✓ It is not carcinogenic (cancer causing) – actually it has been clinically shown to have several anti-cancer effects.

✓ There is no discernable pattern of DNP causing any kind of chronic or serious injury to the human body in all its known history.

✓ All official government claims made in recent times to the effect that DNP is dangerous or injurious to the body are necessarily vague, because there is no specific corroboration for them in the known public record.

✓ If read carefully, virtually all of the official or popularly reported claims against DNP as dangerous, are only referring to the dangers of overdosing or the cataract and rash issues. No matter how much these statements appear to be intended to imply more it is always and only these three reasons they are referring to, because they have no basis for any other claim and so can at best only imply more.

✓ If there is no specific reason for the claims that DNP is dangerous, then everyone voicing them is at best voicing a baseless opinion.

✓ No amount of baseless opinion adds up to anything that should affect public policy; especially for such an efficient, safe and necessary medicine.

✓ The argument that DNP is dangerous because so many medical people make this claim is ridiculous, considering these statements are not based on facts. Whatever the reason for the phenomenon, it is by definition a mass inaccuracy as no one says it for a reason. Whether they are merely repeating other inaccurate statements or their position is skewed by financial or some other personal interest in DNP remaining illegal or they are simply confused by the existing body of unclear and inaccurate statements or some admixture of these causes, what they assert is factually inaccurate.

✓ The danger of overdosing does not amount to a reason to keep this substance from the public, as that would mean virtually every medicine would have to be banned because you can overdose on all of them.

✓ The only reason an effective and needed substance should be banned is because the side effects are unacceptably injurious to the body. This does not apply to overdosing, as that is a universal attribute belonging to all drugs. The only conceivable exception to this, is if a drug can be overdosed at a very low multiple of its minimum effective dose. This is not true of DNP at all. The minimum effective dose is considered 0.6 mg per kg of body weight a day and the minimum fatal dose is estimated by clinicians to be 20-30 mg/kg per day.

The following three statements serve to further simplify and summarize the above line of reasoning.

1. DNP has possibly the greatest benefits of any drug and does no harm unless overdosed or one is allergic.

2. Overdose and allergy are universal attributes, possessed by all drugs. They are not reason to illegalize any valuable drugs.

3. DNP is the most effective therapy for fat reduction known and does not harm the body, giving it possibly the best benefit to side effect ratio of any known medicine. DNP should be a prescription drug.

CHAPTER TWELVE

Answers to Arguments

How can you use a bunch of eighty-year-old information to call into question the wisdom and integrity of the FDA? You weren't there when this all happened, they were.

Not that it's all that critically important, but some of the clinical studies I quote in this book took place over the decades since it was illegalized. Off the top of my head, I would say the most recent I have used was done in the 1980's. As to who was where when, I agree the FDA was in existence during DNP's legal use. They certainly had a better perspective as to how things played out at that time, but that only applies to the FDA then and their decision to ban DNP. The refusal to reverse that decision since that time and the decision to ban DNP in 1938, are two separate and distinct things and I judge them separately.

I do not try to judge the FDA's decision to ban DNP on any reasons they might have had as a result of being there at the time its use was going on legally. I judge that decision on their appallingly insufficient official reason for banning it. Which is *freaking cataracts in one in one thousand women* who used DNP. If there were more and better reasons, they would have given them. They gave that as their sole reason, so I can judge them on it.

As to the refusal to reverse the ban, that is an ongoing behavior even to this very day. Now, unless they have some one-hundred-year-old FDA guy telling them what happened back then, they are working with the same information I am. That available information is the clinical studies and what is known from other use by the public.

Now, that is just what I have been doing up to this point in this book, showing these available historic facts prove that DNP is safe, when not overdosed and is arguably the most important chemical therapy to improve human health and quality of life ever discovered. I think I have shown that the aforementioned available facts fit this contention, but do not support the FDA's actions.

This is the problem with the FDA's position, that the available facts show them to have not only made a terrible decision in banning DNP, but an ongoing and equally bad decision not to reverse it. And in my humble opinion, that initial decision and their failure to reverse it are both so obviously bad, that it was likely they were and are acting in the interest of politically potent special interests, because there is really no other tenable rationale for their acting against the overwhelming interest of the American people. Not to mention, that is exactly what the FDA does for the Pharmaceutical industry, always and incessantly. Is it just me, or is the phrase FDA wisdom and integrity really an oxymoron?

My gosh, DNP is an insecticide and an explosive! You would have to be crazy to eat it!

So, If DNP does no harm to the body, why would it matter what other applications it has? Lots of things we put down our throats have harsh seeming other uses. For instance alcohol has similar uses and attributes but people ingest it like crazy. It's volatile and it is probably used to kill a greater number of life forms than any other substance. Unlike DNP, alcohol *does* harm the body. For instance alcohol harms the liver and DNP doesn't. This argument is like the other arguments against DNP, just a bunch alarmist hype that doesn't stand up to scrutiny.

Are you crazy? DNP is classed as a poison!

DNP's status as a poison is primarily related to its being overdosed and I have covered the logic of that point several times in this book. Anyway, this question begs the another question: whether the government is wrong in claiming that DNP is poisonous or dangerous. This is the central question *and they are the ones trying to give it a bad name.* It is ridiculous to presume the FDA is infallible or objective. The ineptitude and corruptibility of any government agency is a more reasonable presumption. But there is no need to presume either; the truth of the matter is obtained only by looking at the facts.

DNP Killed people that worked around it just because they inhaled it, isn't that poisonous?

This is strictly an overdose issue. DNP can be eaten, absorbed through the skin or inhaled. In each case there will only be a danger if too much is taken in. The men that died probably took in 3 grams or more in a short period by inhalation or through their skin.

This quote from Cutting and Tainters report explains;

> *"Exactly similar effects can be produced in man provided a large enough dose is taken. This was seen occasionally in munition workers during the World War, who absorbed large amounts of dinitrophenol through the lungs or skin."*

You see, they state that it is the large dosage and not the way it is ingested that is dangerous.

Is everyone else wrong and you're right?

No. I am in agreement with virtually all of the clinicians that studied DNP, in that that they considered it essentially safe and indispensable for treating obesity. So, I agree with them. Since nobody has a specific claim of negative side effects that would be sufficient to ban such a valuable medicine, at least in that sense, I am in agreement with almost everyone else. I disagree with the FDA, and everyone that follows their lead, in what the facts add up to. I just read the facts the same way the DNP clinicians did. The FDA and their adherents simply hype and re-characterize the facts to suit their preconceptions or interests. These preconceptions are based on the accumulated confusion brought about by years of obscurity and misrepresentation and are ultimately attributable to self-interest.

The reality is, that there is no financial incentive for any particular individual or entity to push for legalization of DNP. There is a *HUGE* financial incentive for certain large and powerful special interests to keep DNP an illegal substance. *Consequently you get an official position heavily slanted in favor of those large and powerful special interests by their female dog, the FDA. This in turn decides virtually everyone else's position.*

Why does the 1934 Stanford report that you rely on so heavily say DNP should only be used as a last resort?

The short answer is, that the political pressure against DNP had become so intense, that the three Stanford clinicians that had released this report said one or two erratic and inconsistent things under the duress of that pressure, while still maintaining an overwhelmingly positive position on DNP.

Whether they were directly and personally pressured is not known, but likely they were. That report carefully analyzed their various study's results, other clinical studies and everything known about DNP from the first year of public use. Two facts are beyond question. They asserted clearly and often that DNP was by far the most

> "Whether they were directly and personally pressured is not known, but likely they were."

effective drug for fat reduction; and the only truly negative side effect they found was the fairly low occurrence allergic skin rash reaction.

That is the short answer, but this question is so important it is worthwhile to go into considerable detail to prove their true position on DNP in that report. More specifically, that though they said it, they clearly did not believe DNP should be a last resort only therapy. This is a bold sounding claim, but it is really an understatement. Lets go through the pertinent statements from that report and see:

First they assert DNP's incredible effectiveness throughout the document; here are just a few quotes;

> *"Our experimental results and those of all other investigators are in essential agreement on the remarkable powers of dinitrophenol for augmenting oxidative metabolism by a direct action on the tissues or cells."*

> *"It can now be said that dinitrophenolnis of definite value as a drug for treating obesity and perhaps some other metabolic disorders".*

> *"In a preliminary report on the loss of body weight in obese individuals, it was stated that losses of to 3 pounds a week could be obtained with doses of dinitrophenol which were well tolerated. Three other groups of workers have confirmed this result in smaller groups of patients, and it is now a common experience with many practicing physicians."*

> *"However, this will in no way affect the great significance of dinitrophenol as having been the first foreign agent, or drug, to be demonstrated as a very potent and well nigh universal metabolic stimulant, which was available for experimental purposes and useful for alleviation of human infirmity".*

Now a partial list of the clear and highly specific assertions that DNP does not harm patients in any way as long as it is properly dosed: (The one exception being, that some people have an allergic reaction).

FATAL EFFECTS

They point out that while DNP can be fatally overdosed it happened only two times in the first year with over 100,000 people using it for extended periods of time and many without doctor supervision. Here is how they characterize this fact,

> *"When one considers that some one hundred thousand patients have been treated with this exceedingly potent therapeutic agent, it is a matter of some gratification to know that fatalities have not been more numerous."*

They then go over possible negative effects on the body, organ by organ, and conclude:

1. DNP definitely does not harm the liver.

2. DNP does not harm the kidneys.

3. DNP does not even affect the circulation, which is a huge benefit and unique to this metabolic stimulant. There is no change in blood pressure. It actually helps people with high blood pressure, by bringing it down as they lose fat.

4. Blood- They discuss a lot on this issue but the bottom line is that it has no harmful effects on the blood.

5. Cardiovascular System- They state quite clearly and specifically, that DNP does not harm or even affect the pulse. They say this makes DNP unique among other thermogenics.

6. Heart- They are emphatic that DNP does not harm the heart.

GASTROINTESTINAL TRACT –Here are their own words on this point;

> *"The claim that this drug is a severe irritant to the gastrointestinal tract of patients is unwarranted for doses of therapeutic range, according to our experience*

and to that of large numbers of physicians prescribing it."

So the three clinicians have come up with a skin rash allergic side effect, that a small percentage of users get and nothing more. By the way, most prescription drugs have a skin rash allergic reaction for some people.

They report no other damage or injury to the body of any kind. With such a highly detailed and specific report, it is unimaginable that they did know of some specific danger and just didn't bother to mention it.

But in spite of all this, they go on to make two statements that sound somewhat negative about DNP. One is understandable but the other one is almost irrational, in view of everything else they say in the document.

The somewhat negative but understandable statement is;

> *"This problem is particularly pressing since 'obesity cures' are extensively bought by fat people for self-medication without diagnosis. Therefore, it would seem desirable that dinitrophenol be added to the poison list, and its sale regulated so it could not be obtained except on a physician's prescription".*

The bad sounding part is that they recommend DNP should be placed on the "poison list" this sounds pretty bad, except that they follow that suggestion in the same sentence with the assertion that it should be allowed as a prescription medicine. So, they are not saying it is poisonous in the sense that it is deadly or harmful. They want it put on the poison list, because they want it to be a prescription medicine only. Apparently, putting DNP on the poison list, was the most expedient way to make it a prescription only drug. So this statement is not so much negative, as it is slightly confusing because of the terminology.

This is the sort of line DNP's enemies will take out of context to undermine the real meaning of this document. This is why I bothered to point out the obvious here.

The second negative statement is just plain irrational, when placed in the context of the rest of the document. Ultimately, I believe that very fact proves to support my position regarding DNP, when it is analyzed a little closer and in the context of the rest of the document. Here is the statement in question:

> *"Certainly, it should not be used as a routine measure in any clinical condition. Obesity can be controlled in most cases by the physician who will patiently supervise the dietary regime. In other cases, thyroid or thyroxine may be needed. It is only when all other measures have been thoroughly tried and found ineffective, and when there is impelling need for weight reduction, that dinitrophenol medication, with a knowledge of attending risks, should be undertaken. Under these circumstances, the physician must balance the prospective benefit against the potential harm, just as he does with any therapeutic procedure, and give the patient his best chance. This summary of the clinical effects and side actions of dinitrophenol shows that in some respects this drug is not ideal as a therapeutic agent, since it may cause certain undesired side-actions in a portion of the patients treated. However, this does not mean that it cannot be used safely under proper conditions."*

So far, they have stated that DNP is the most effective fat reduction therapy known.

Then they have asserted that it is safe and well tolerated at therapeutic doses. Then, they go into great detail explaining and proving organ-by-organ and system-by-system, that DNP is harmless.

They also state that it has a very low occurrence of fatal overdose giving it an advantage over many other drugs regarding that risk.

They ultimately come up with one side effect, an allergic rash. A rash allergy is common to a great many drugs as well as many other things. This would never be a reason to make an incredibly effective drug, a therapy of last resort only. From a side effects standpoint, having found only one minor allergic reaction after such extensive clinical study and popular use is as good as it gets for any drug.

In spite of all this they say: *"Certainly, it should not be used as a routine measurein any clinical condition."*

Then, they schizophrenically return to saying DNP is safe, ending the same paragraph with this: *"However, this does not mean that it cannot be used safely under proper conditions".*

So immediately after saying that DNP should not be used as a routine clinical measure, they say it can be used safely.

To add to the mystery, they discuss the possibility of discovering another compound, that will ultimately replace DNP in effectiveness, while being free of negative side effects, when the only negative side effect they have discovered is a skin rash. There are not very many drugs with only one or two allergic reactions and nothing else. So it is absurd to hold out for something that doesn't even have that side effect.

They end the report with the following sentence:

"However, this will in no way affect the great significance of dinitrophenol as having been the first foreign agent, or drug, to be demonstrated as a very potent and well nigh universal metabolic stimulant, which was available for experimental purposes and useful for alleviation of human infirmity".

This is the highest possible praise for DNP. Saying that it is the first effective drug for fat reduction, means it is the only one, because they had just discovered it a year before and just stated that perhaps some new compounds will be discovered.

Then they elevate DNP to heroic status in saying it is *"well nigh universal metabolic stimulant,"* The three clinicians tip their hat by ending their document with this over the top high praise. This is not consistent with saying DNP should be a drug of last resort.

So how do we explain this erratic and illogical discourse? The enemies of this book and of DNP will say that it is obvious that even the Clinicians that I quote as supporting my contentions, either disagree with me or are at least ambivalent. The problem is that this contention does not hold up to scrutiny. With just a little analysis, it becomes obvious that this could not possibly be the case. For the sake of brevity, I will just give a very condensed version of one such proof.

Why did they not list anywhere in this document at least one sufficiently harmful effect, that was the reason DNP should be a last resort drug? They have only given allergic skin rash. Since this is not reason enough to explain make it a drug of last resort only, the only other possibilities are that they either hid some harmful side effect or somehow intuited one. It is ridiculous to think they hid something and there is no hint of any such danger anywhere else in the public record, except for the soon to be discovered cataract issue. If they had some amorphous foreboding weighing on them regarding DNP, they have given absolutely no fact or pattern of effects to support it anywhere in the report. Anyway, this is not the way clinicians approach data, they deal in empirical facts and that is certainly the case with this document throughout. So we either have to dismiss the rest of the document or that one statement. There is no way it makes sense to dismiss all of their assertions because of this statement.

We are still left with the fact that the clincians did say it should not be routinely used, juxtaposed with the fact that nothing can be found to support that position in their report. As a matter of fact, almost every assertion and fact in the report supports the opposite position; that it should be used often because of its incredible efficacy and exceptional harmlessness.

Also, if you notice, they surround the last resort statement with assertions that totally undermine and disprove it. These pro-DNP statements and the fact that they immediately proceed and follow the anti-DNP statement show, that they could not bring themselves to truly maintain that DNP should be a last resort therapy, because they immediately undermine the statement.

So, if they didn't believe it why did they say it? They give us a little hint at the beginning of the report when in the very first sentence they say: *"The interest in and enthusiasm for this product were so great that its widespread use has become a matter of some concern in public health"*.

So they are in part writing this report to respond to some public or official concern. To get a better idea of the exact source and nature of that concern here is a statement from an FDA document.

> *"In August 1934, the Food and Drug Administration issued the first of a series of warnings, pointing out that sales of dinitrophenol fat reducers were booming, despite the reports of deaths, but the 1906 Food and Drugs Act did not cover products of this type. All FDA could do was to warn the public."...Nevertheless, the agency was preparing for action -- to test the law if nothing else."*

The FDA released this warning one month before this Stanford DNP report was released. So the Clinicians and their highly successful work with DNP were under full-scale attack from the FDA. When you put it in that context, it makes a lot more sense that the three Stanford Clinicians would at least attempt to make some small concession to that fact. While this alone would explain this statement, I think there is a little more here than meets the eye. They were almost certainly getting some pressure themselves to promote the idea that DNP had too many negatives to be of real value. They fell short of saying that, but they did cave in enough to perhaps mollify the Stanford University board of directors, the AMA or whoever it was that had been pressured to put pressure on them. The great reluctance they had towards making the statement is shown by the fact that they are so quick to state the opposite in the very next sentence. If they were reluctant but still did so, it is almost certain there was outside pressure of some sort.

To whatever extent you agree or disagree with this book's contentions, for the sake of analysis, take as a given that DNP is truly safe and effective. It follows as a certainty, that some individual or group had some self-interested motivation to stop the use of DNP. The only other possibility is that it was all a misunderstanding, which makes sense for the public at large and many who unwittingly worked in government to ban DNP, but cannot explain the fact that there was a strong unrelenting push against it. That a misunderstanding based on two overdose deaths and some allergic rashes could weather all of the resistance and scrutiny such a ban would face, makes no sense at all. Such a misunderstanding could not supply sufficient impetuous and fortitude to carry through the process of banning such a beneficial medicine. There are many other obvious reasons that misunderstanding could not be the only cause of the ban, but I will give just two:

First, at some point the people interested in keeping DNP legal would put up enough resistance to force the well intentioned, but mistaken officials to advert to the facts enough to see their blatantly obvious mistake.

Second, if you look at the public record of FDA claims, there is a clear pattern of a smear campaign, that just could not be perpetrated as a simple mistake, the literary tactics are transparently disingenuous, to the point of being laughably smarmy.

For the ban process to continue with such inexorable and focused determination, there must have been someone motivated by more than just confusion. Most likely, it was several people that had sufficient financial and political resources to push the ban through. The most likely culprit is the pharmaceutical industry. They had a lot to lose if DNP wasn't banned and they are the entity that has developed a symbiotic relationship with the FDA.

What we are most likely looking at here is the nascent genesis of the present day cabal that the FDA and pharmaceutical companies have become. The pharmaceutical companies have obscene profit margins that outstrip any other industry by far. This is due to the role the FDA plays in providing and protecting the monopoly the pharmaceutical companies presently enjoy. This is particularly disgusting, considering that medical healing is so necessary to human happiness and the government is supposed to protect the interest of its citizens. Instead, both parties work against their natural calling in headlong pursuit of profit and power. DNP is the first, the greatest and most egregious instance of this evil dynamic. Avarice is indeed the root of all evil and has become the essential reason and purpose for the FDA's existence.

Ok let's say your assertion that the financial interests' of powerful industries explain DNPs remaining a banned substance. Why does the FDA want to keep it banned? They have no financial incentive.

Well, in an ideal world that would be true. The FDA should act in the interest of the American public. The reality is that all concentrations of governmental power are, to some extent, manipulated for the financial gain of a few and against the interest of the many. Even if the FDA had no financial interest, it is still heavily lobbied and pressured, at least indirectly all the time. But the FDA does have a financial interest. It receives a huge percentage of its funding directly from the pharmaceutical companies. The FDA charges a fee to process the application for new drugs that can cost as much as five hundred thousand dollars per drug application. One expert compares this to the mafia paying the FBI a fee for services.

The nature and finality of the FDA's decision-making ability has *HUGE* financial ramifications for these pharmaceutical companies. Billions and billions of dollars rise and fall on its caprice and fiat. This incestuous relationship serves as a cabal. The FDA employees get power and jobs through the profits of the pharmaceutical companies. If you really look at the facts, it becomes obvious that the FDA exists to limit all forms of competition to the pharmaceutical companies as much as possible.

So pervasive is this manipulation of the FDA, that Dr. Herbert Lay, after three years as FDA commissioner, resigned as head of that corrupt bureaucracy in exasperation. At the time he expressed his disgust to the San Francisco Chronicle saying, "The thing that bugs me is that people think the FDA is protecting them. It isn't. What the FDA is doing and what the public thinks its doing are as different as night and day." (January 2, 1970).

Now that's a man who ran the FDA. He was at the top, he knows. But really, did you need him to tell you that? Are government and corruption not often virtually synonymous? The FDA is standing between the fat loss industry and its extinction. You don't think that industry wouldn't spend billions if necessary to influence the decision to keep DNP shelved? To the degree that anyone at the FDA leaned towards legalizing DNP, they would be shut down by pressure from more sophisticated and cynical higher ups; either because they saw the writing on the wall or because pressure was put on them from the weight loss or medical industries that understandably feel financially threatened by DNP. It's simple, greed and ignorance are winning and the American people are losing and the FDA is not going to help.

What if there is something they don't know yet, some unknown danger to DNP?

You could say that about anything, from aspirin to newly approved medicines. Clinicians who did extensive large scale testing called it "well tolerated at therapeutic doses and indispensable." If something is later discovered that makes it unacceptable then, like anything else, it should be removed.

Why should we listen to you rather than the FDA?

I am not saying to listen to me. Listen to the clinicians who knew DNP better than anyone. They wanted to keep it a prescription medicine. They thought it safe and indispensable. Listen to them. Also, listen to facts and reason. The facts say that it is safe. Reason and facts tell us that it is as valuable as any medicine, because it is the perfect solution to the greatest health problem. You should not listen to me, but you should listen to my arguments, insofar as they are reasonable and supported by the facts and experts.

Also, it is a matter of record that the FDA is in the pocket of the pharmaceutical industry. For instance, many politicians, including congressman Henry Waxman and Senator Charles Grassley, have often asserted that the FDA is corrupted by the pharmaceutical industry and primarily serves that industry's interest. It has been proven in court as well. Just read the FDA Fun Facts chapter for a sampling of what is written and said on this issue. Whoever you listen to it definitely should not be the FDA.

Why should I listen to you rather than my doctor?

Same answer as above. Anyway, doctors are often wrong, they're human. Listen to the clinical doctors, who were experts on DNP, instead of your doctor who is at best vaguely aware of the hype against it. Besides, you should read all the scandals that come from the relationship between many doctors and the pharmaceutical industry. Google it, It's shocking. If you read up on that, you will realize, that as with any other walk of life, self-interest reins supreme. Many doctors are just not objective.

You're just trying to make money on this.

Well, I did write a book for the purpose of publication. One of my motivations is to get some reimbursement for my efforts. But it does not follow that I am untruthful about my true opinions to others or myself. There is a way to tell whether I am in earnest or not. Just take a look at my research, reasoning and proofs for my position on DNP. It becomes obvious that I am in earnest, as I have made an overwhelmingly strong case. In my opinion my case is airtight. Heck, I am even making all of the best arguments against my own position and answering them. If I were disingenuous I would be vague and indulge in innuendo, as I would be holding a position for personal gain and not because it was factual or true (kind of like many of those who want to keep DNP in mothballs). The reality is, that this is a crusade against injustice that I feel keenly about.

One other thing, if making money was my primary motivation, I would not push the fact that DNP is such a financial threat to so many, that it ought to be legalized and that greed is keeping it from us. These assertions will only serve to alarm and motivate those who feel financially threatened by DNP and the truth about it contained in my book.

I honestly believe, that to the degree this book gains popular recognition, there will be an attempt to undermine it and silence me. That's what large interests with resources do, when their industries and profits are threatened. It is inevitable. I don't care, bring it. I hate seeing so many people deprived of something they need so desperately because of selfishness, greed and ignorance. So, if this were just or even primarily for money, I would only discuss how effective and safe DNP was and not antagonize my new enemies.

138

Even body builders say that DNP is a dangerous and harsh substance.

It's ironic that the much of the community that has brought DNP use back from obscurity are also the same people that are giving it a bad name. I first found out about DNP from reading the boards and forums of these folks. My early impressions of DNP were all negative due to my body builder forum research. Like so many of those in the body building community, who had never used DNP, I thought it was a dangerous and harsh substance used only by extreme risk takers.

But it was from reading their DNP use logs that I first began to suspect the truth that DNP is neither harsh nor dangerous. I noticed a pattern. First, all of the body builders that had the most negative view of DNP were the ones that never used it. It is this crowd of body builders, who have no personal experience, that perpetuates the myth that DNP is one of the more dangerous substances used in bodybuilding. The ones that did use it, almost always made statements that DNP was a harsh experience and something to be taken seriously. But, when you read their actual cycle logs they really only ever complained about the side effects that were due to overdosing e.g. lethargy, sweating etc. Nobody ever claimed to be hurt by his or her DNP use, just that it was unpleasant to use it.

The next thing I realized was that DNP use for body builders is often an unpleasant experience, due only to the fact that they overdose it. The reason they overdose it is due to the nature of their profession or sport. When body builders go through a "bulking phase" to gain massive amounts of muscle, they consume a huge volume of calories a day. When they are done with this process, they have gained some fat as well. It is imperative to lose this fat quickly because they lose muscle also during that process. This is especially true at the pro level where they need to be as massively muscular as possible with body fat percentages as low as possible. For this reason, they majorly overdose DNP, often consuming amounts in ten days, that they should take over a twenty or thirty-day period. The side effects are completely from intense fat burning induced heat and those are the *only* complaints I have found.

Some people have an allergic reaction. (Rash, cataracts)

Do I really have to answer this? Ok, let's ban antibiotics because some people are allergic. As a matter of fact, let's get rid of pretty much everything you can put in your mouth because there are people with an allergic reaction for just about everything.

OOORR

How about we give the allergic people antihistamines, and if there are a few that still get a rash, they just don't take it, if they dislike the rash more than being fat. Then, everyone else takes DNP and gets healthy and beautiful, while simultaneously wiping out the weight-loss industry! Personally, I'm a plan B guy, but that's just me. * (The same goes for the much rarer cataract reaction.)

If what you're saying is all true, then DNP would be legal.

No. If just one half of what I'm saying is true, it would be legal; the half that says DNP's benefits are without equal and it is safe, if used properly. Unfortunately, the other half about greed and ignorance is also true and that explains DNP's legal status.

Even if everything you're saying is true, people would abuse it by purposefully overeating and taking DNP instead of leading healthy lives.

I agree that DNP could be used liike a Roman vomitorium in a pill. I would be against that. Such behavior would be little more than gluttony or medicinal bulimia. But the fact that some people would abuse something is not a reason for its being made illegal. If its benefits are great enough, it should be allowed. Take the opiate family of painkillers like Vicodin® for example. Many do abuse them. But, who for that reason, would say they should be entirely removed from the market leaving people in serious pain with no relief?

If what you're saying is true, then DNP is immoral because it's too easy. People should just quit overeating and diet and exercise.

To begin with, many people are overweight or obese for glandular, hormonal or other medical conditions. Many others have an over-efficient metabolism (their bodies use and conserve energy very efficiently) or possess constitutions that for a variety of reasons make it extremely difficult, if not virtually impossible, to keep excess fat off. If for no other reason, it should be a prescription medicine for all of these kinds of people.

The morality-gluttony argument against DNP regarding everyone else who does not fall into these categories is still worth discussing. In my opinion, this kind of hard-hearted thinking gives religion and morality a bad name.

Take a woman who is fifty pounds overweight, having a normal metabolism. She got that way by being a sedentary stay at home mom and consuming more calories than she burnt off over a period of ten years. That's five pounds a year, not exactly profligate gluttony. People who find themselves in this situation rarely have the necessary combination of time, constitution, health and will power to exercise and diet to get the fat off. It is the rare exception that a person removes this unwanted fat that has crept up over the years and is now threatening their health and undermining their happiness. Now, if a few months of DNP treatment makes them thin again, they have a second chance. All they need to do is eat a maintenance calorie diet. This is something many of these people could and would do, people who would not have done the one or two years of rigorous dieting and exercise to get thin. Now tell me, is that immoral? No, it's not by anyone's standards.

But let's say some of those women, after getting thin, were to continue to overeat and take DNP to stay thin in a chronic and abusive way. I would not be in favor of that. But they would be doing the wrong thing with or without DNP, because they are chronic gluttons and that is what's wrong, not being thin. So you see, keeping DNP from those who find themselves in need of it, even if it is partly their own fault, just to make sure nobody gets away with anything is just self-righteous, petty, and negativistic emoting. It is not religion, morality or a zeal for public health.

Now, I can see other questions that I have not answered specifically enough to quiet the excessively harsh and judgmental tendencies of some people. But with people like that, such an effort is in my experience, an exercise in futility. For all but the hardest of heart, this question has been more than adequately answered.

You're just a conspiracy monger.

No, I really don't think that way actually. I'm just not a "black helicopter" guy. I don't think there is a truly organized effort to hide the truth about DNP. What I do believe is that greed is playing a decisive role in keeping DNP in mothballs. The clinical studies and extensive public use show the truth, that DNP is a perfect solution to the weight loss problem. Now, you would think medical associations and pharmaceutical companies would see this and bring DNP back to the aid of the American people. But the reality is, that DNP is ignored or even to some extent purposely misrepresented.

Here is how greed manifests itself, as well as the dominant role self interest takes, as the manipulation of government plays out in a rather passive way. To the extent anyone working in the weight-loss or pharmaceutical industries takes a look at DNP and suspects the truth, they are faced with at least some sense of the financial ramifications. Now, unless they have a financial incentive or some other kind of self-interested gain to pursue legalization of DNP, they are unlikely to follow through on any such effort, because it would be a costly and uphill battle.

This is presuming of course, that we are speaking of someone who is in a position to actually mount a serious attempt to change DNP's legal status. For instance, take a man who is president of a major pharmaceutical company. If he became aware that DNP was really the most needed medicine in existence, the more he looked into DNP, the more he would realize that it would wipe all of his company's fat loss products and do severe damage to many of his company's other partiality related medication sales.

For example, if his company produced a line of heart related products like cholesterol drugs, sale of such drugs would drop off tremendously, if everyone were able to become thin. This man would have some idea of the damage to his company's bottom line. Let's say, for the sake of illustration, he estimated a loss of 30% or roughly a billion a year in profit.

To add to the difficulty, his company would get no help, but instead tremendous resistance from the rest of the industry. So his company would bear the risk and expense alone, to get a product legalized, that could not be patented. Now, since DNP cannot be patented, it cannot be monopolized. This means the price couldn't be kept high. This man would know that even if he somehow got DNP legalized, every other pharmaceutical company would be making it as well. Since DNP is dirt-cheap and there would be open market competition, there is no real upside for this man or his company. Even if he had the intelligence and honesty to see the truth and the altruism to risk losing his job to do the right thing, he probably wouldn't even consider it, because he would know it would be absolutely hopeless. As good men so often do, such an individual would most likely stoically accept the human condition with its manifold injustices, without even mentioning it to anyone. But, if he did try, he would without question, be rejected as stupid and dangerous and not a company man. This same scenario applies to anyone in the government or the medical industry. Now that is not a conspiracy theory, it's called common sense about human nature and the way the world really works. Anyway, how else do you explain the present situation with DNP, in spite of the fact that it is clinically proven safe, effective and perhaps the most valuable medicine known to man?

How could a conspiracy of the large scale that you're claiming be kept secret?

To begin with, I do not think this is a large-scale conspiracy, in the sense that a lot of people in the FDA and other government agencies are *fully consciously* complicit in hiding the truth about DNP. I will explain my understanding of how DNP was made the object of a misinformation campaign back when it was originally banned. How it is kept banned is attributable to DNP's illegal status, the general public's ignorance of its existence, and the momentum of the misinformation campaign perpetrated against it.

From 1933 to 1934, DNP had its first year of legal use in the USA. The experience that people had with it was amazing. It melted fat off their bodies at a tremendous rate, in the same manner that exercise does. The only known negative side effect, other than the harmless ones shared with exercise, was that a small percentage of people would develop an allergic reaction in the form of a skin rash. We can be sure of this fact, from the Stanford report released in 1934, that covered the extensive human and animal studies done at that University, as well as other clinical studies around the world. This report also covered what was known from the vast prescription and non-prescription use by the American public that year.

So, a miracle fat reduction drug had been discovered, which was safe and incredibly effective. In spite of this, at the very time this report was released, the FDA was already trying to suppress this medical breakthrough (DNP). This fact is alluded to in this same report and also more recently, it is more specifically stated in an FDA published document, both are found in this book.

If the Stanford clinicians could find no harm in DNP from their vast personal direct experience, as well as their understanding of the public record regarding DNP, where was the FDA getting their information? The FDA does no clinical studies on its own. The FDA relies completely on external clinical studies. The FDA was looking at the same body of information as the Stanford clinicians and coming up with exactly the opposite conclusion. The reason is that the source of this conclusion of the FDA was not objective information, but pressure from the people that were being financially threatened by DNP.

In this situation, the true conspirators are the people that used money, lobbyists and any other political entrenchments they possessed to achieve their ends. This could have been a very small number of top executives at a few large pharmaceutical companies. While these men knew that their motivation was financial, they would not reveal that information, while pushing to illegalize DNP. They would assert that their motivation was simply that DNP was dangerous.

These same people would have financed a misinformation campaign to promote this lie as well. They would have gotten experts to lend credibility to the position that DNP was dangerous; most likely utilizing doctors employed by their own companies. If necessary, they would have pressured or even bribed government officials including FDA officials.

Most likely, there were a few doctors, FDA officials and other government officials, that had a pretty good idea of what was going on.

Whether anyone in the FDA was explicitly aware that they were serving special interests, rather than public interests, doesn't really matter. What does matter is that the further down the chain of authority, and the further away from the real conspirators, the less aware people would be of this fact. In other words, most of the people

145

that played a role in pushing for DNP to be illegalized were either partially or completely ignorant of the truth. They were either completely duped or partially so and simply following orders to keep their jobs.

It is logical and common knowledge that this is normal behavior for the FDA. Countless doctors, politicians, FDA whistle blowers have said this and it has been proven in court. The FDA primarily serves the interests of the large pharmaceutical companies and of course, that involves a few people deceiving the public. I am sure they are always careful to keep as few people as possible privy to the truth, when they do this. This dynamic is really common sense, but since I am dealing with a "big lie" it is necessary to cover all of the bases, even the relatively obvious ones, to inoculate people as much as possible against the propaganda machine that will be employed against this book's message. It is an unfortunate reality that those who have the reins of power and authority, or even just popular opinion on their side, can so easily confuse and deceive so many, with so little effort.

Your comparison in the prolog to antibiotics is overly dramatic and not apt, because antibiotics are lifesaving and there is no real replacement for them. There are lots of ways for people to lose weight and they don't die from it all that often.

Wrong. More people die from complications from obesity than anything else. It just takes longer to kill them. Excess fat causes more sorrow, suffering and death than infection would, even without antibiotics. I won't even bother to quote statistics. If you don't believe me, either Google it yourself or better yet, just take a walk at the mall and look around you.

As to diet and exercise being a solution for many, that's true. But there are some who it would not work for. But even for the many who could lose weight that way, it is just too difficult and people are

146

rarely successful. Either way you look at it, the analogy to antibiotics is apt because obesity is the top killer, as well as the cause of manifold sufferings. If anything, the antibiotics comparison is a bit of an understatement. It is difficult to wrap our minds around the immense scale of the ramifications of this FDA treachery, but seeing that it is worse than if antibiotics were taken from us, helps.

Why do you hate and distrust the weight loss and medical industries?

I don't hate either one, and I don't distrust the weight loss industry any more than any other industry. I just know enough about human nature and the sad role greed and self-interest often play in human affairs. These two industries just happen to be comprised entirely of humans. I am simply reacting to what I consider to be their destructive, selfish and unjust behavior in this matter.

However, I do distrust the medical/pharmaceutical industries probably more than any other. They use the government, especially the FDA with its vast regulatory powers, to maintain an iron-fisted monopoly over American health care. They keep prices artificially high and have created an artificially elite economic class. Unfortunately, for the doctors though, the insurance industry has in recent decades moved in and hijacked the whole scam away from them. Now most doctors make a mere fraction of their formerly top salary among professional's income.

The insurance companies achieved this impressive feat of stealing from the thieves by gaining control of the revenue stream and subsequently leveraging that ultimate power position to negotiate all of the profits back to themselves. This gives a whole new meaning to the old saying, "everyone hates the middle man."

Maybe, I should distrust the insurance companies even more than the medical industry.

The only consolation for the doctors is that now the insurance companies have to deal with the voracious pack of lawyers; keeping them at bay by giving them a big slice of their overpriced ill-gotten pie. Perhaps, I should distrust the lawyers more than anyone. Under any circumstance, from a financial standpoint it sure sucks to be sick or even to be healthy, if you have medical insurance.

My Questions to Those Still in Doubt

It is the position of the FDA that DNP is extremely poisonous and dangerous to human health. Why is their position totally at odds with the human clinical studies done on DNP, where no such dangers were found? The same is true with the legal use by the public for five years; also with the modern day underground use, and my own personal experience with DNP. Here are my questions to those who still doubt as to whether DNP is truly safe and effective.

- ❖ If DNP is not safe, for reasons other than overdosing or rare allergic reactions, why is there no specific record of those claims anywhere?

- ❖ Since there are no specific claims that DNP damages or injures any part of the body, what excuse is there for banning it?

- ❖ Why did the clinicians at Stanford University, who did the most extensive human clinical studies of DNP done in this country and also prescribed it to thousands of people a year, say that it was well tolerated at therapeutic doses?

- ❖ Why didn't those same clinicians find anything other than the risk of a skin rash allergy?

- ❖ Why did those clinicians specifically describe the various systems and organs of the body that DNP did no harm to, and never once mention any part of the body it did harm?

- ❖ Why did they specifically point out, that in spite of the fact that there were no controls on a huge amount of public use, that there was an incredibly small percentage of fatal overdose and why did they say it was a reason for gratification? Doesn't this prove, that it is not an easily overdosed medicine?

- ❖ Why did they suggest DNP remain a prescription medicine?

- ❖ Why did the FDA only site a rare allergic reaction (cataracts) and overdosing as the reasons for banning it?

- ❖ If the FDA had other or better reasons, why did they not mention them?

- ❖ Why is it not obvious that the fact that the FDA did not mention any other harmful effects definitive proof that they had no other reason to ban it?

- ❖ Why are so many drugs that do harm the kidneys, liver, heart etc. legally prescribed, when DNP, which does not have those negative side effects, *is* banned for an incredibly rare allergic reaction?

- ❖ Why do people not look at these facts objectively, instead of closing their minds and assuming the ban of DNP must be for good reason, when it is common knowledge, that the pharmaceutical companies and the FDA are not at all trustworthy?

- ❖ Do they think that anyone that resists DNP being a prescription drug, even though they do it for no reason they can point to, must be right somehow?

- ❖ Do they think everyone against DNP is spontaneously intuiting some unknown danger?

- ❖ Why are so many people so stubborn and dense when faced with the facts?

CHAPTER THIRTEEN

Changing the Legal Status (USA)

In my opinion, there is almost no chance of DNP being legalized, but that is no reason not to try. This book is, among other things, my initiation of an effort to do that very thing. If there is anyone, who would be in favor of making an organized effort of some kind, I would possibly be interested in helping. Here is what such a movement would be up against.

> **FACT: Obesity increases the risk of osteoarthritis and gynecological problems such as infertility.**
> http://www.cdc.gov/nccdphp/dnpa/obesit

The forces that would be arrayed against such an effort would have virtually unlimited financial resources. The entire weight loss industry would be fighting for its very existence. They would be willing to spend whatever amount necessary to keep DNP from seeing the light of day. Think about it, if DNP became a prescription medicine, why would anyone need Jenny Craig®? Admittedly, eating healthy would still be important, but you can eat healthy without a weight loss company. Those companies just help you control caloric intake, without having to pay attention to your calorie count.

Liposuction? I don't think so! Too violent, expensive and dangerous of a surgery for most anyone to pay for and endure the pain and risks involved, with DNP available. The same is true with gastric bypass. The benefit-risk-discomfort ratio of that rather brutal and sometimes deadly procedure is no comparison to DNP. Here is a question that the FDA really owes the American people an answer to: Why do you continue to ban DNP, but you allow liposuction and gastric bypass? Those two surgeries take far more lives and cause far more suffering and side effects than DNP would, even if it was as bad as you say or at least, imply it is. But DNP isn't harmful and it is so effective, it would make those two brutal procedures that you do allow, to become obsolete.

Other weight loss medications? Why would anyone spend money on any existing drug out there? Either they don't work or are barely effective. DNP works fast and for everyone and is probably safer than anything else that is even remotely effective.

While you may not have thought about these things, those financially threatened by DNP will think of this anytime they are faced with it. When most people first heard of mp3s they thought, "cool, free music!" On the other hand, record storeowners were terrified. They viewed MP3s as a threat to their livelihood. They would have spent everything they could to eradicate MP3 technology. They were unable to stem that tide, because the genie-out-of-the-bottle nature of that technology made that impossible. Now, MP3s have become the mainstream media for music. I promise you, people and organizations in the weight loss industry, will see the writing on the wall and act decisively.

At first, they will ignore this book and hope it doesn't gain any traction in the public consciousness. Then, if it starts to get attention, they will try to undermine both my credibility and the credibility of my book.

If something like an organized effort to legalize DNP were to spring up, these companies would spend whatever they had to on lawyers, political lobbyists and a misinformation campaign to stop the dreaded, evil, poisonous DNP and its lunatic proponents.

The same is true of the medical industry. Both doctors and pharmaceutical companies would take a huge hit to their gross dollar volume. Just to throw a number out there, say 30 percent. You see, a huge percentage of their income is due to poor health from extra body fat and they know it. Now, I am not saying that all doctors are greedy.

I am saying that human nature has that selfish side, and this would manifest itself in the case of DNP legalization, just like any other case. (Since the FDA is basically the medical industry's female dog, what do you think the chances are of FDA changing their position?)

For example, any doctor that defended DNP would be seen as a traitor and be spurned as a quack. This already happens to many doctors who promote natural or unconventional treatments. Most people will not stand up to the wrath of their peers to defend principle, especially to undermine their own self-interest. For the most part, doctors would not even look into DNP. They would go along with the party line. Most people quickly choose the easy path of self-interested ignorance, without even a cursory glance toward the truth. Admit it, you know that's true.

You would not only have a desperate and countless tide of foes with virtually depthless pockets, but you would have an almost impossible task in trying to educate the public about the truth.

All the anti-DNP crowd would have to do is shout things like "deadly," "death," "poison," "cataracts," "liver damage," "kidney damage," etc.

Proponents of DNP would have to carefully make an information intensive argument, to both the public and the FDA. I won't even try to discuss the difficulties of trying to educate the public, it's just too depressing.

The FDA is another matter. It's the FDA's job to weigh the benefits and risks of potential therapies like DNP. This, they have already decided wrongly, and they will never change that decision for all of the reasons already mentioned. All we can expect them to do, is to continue to protect an essentially obsolete weight loss industry and the gross dollar volume of the medical industry. After all, these two industries and the pharmaceutical industry, that sits astride both, have the money, lobbyists and other political entrenchments to use the FDA to keep the banned status of DNP.

The only way I could realistically see that DNP could return to its former status as a legal prescription medicine, is if some wealthy elite or a large organized effort were to finance new clinical studies and a very expensive public information campaign. This would still not achieve much without tremendous public pressure on politicians. Then, you would see a real media battle over the truth, between the public interest and the special interests aligned against DNP.

Even then, it would be a long shot. It would almost have to become part of the platform of one of the two major political parties. If that happened, the party that included it in its platform would have a huge advantage politically. There are a lot of people desperate for a solution to their weight problems. Most people are at least vaguely aware that the FDA is not their friend and would like to see them put in their place.

The focus and opportunity created by DNP legalization being a part of one of the two major political party's platforms, would almost guarantee it being justly and victoriously returned to the American people. That would give me immense personal satisfaction. I hate the way that greed and ignorance usually prevails in circumstances of this kind. The American people are really being wronged in an unusually terrible way in this matter.

CHAPTER FOURTEEN

Part One Final Word

This book has kept its promise. I have proven that DNP is the most effective fat reduction therapy known. I have also proven that DNP has no known harmful effects at therapeutic doses, that are sufficient reason to ban it. Along with these two truths, I have also shown that there is no good reason to keep this vital medicine from the American people.

It is a sad reality, that greed and self-interest stand between the American people and this most needed of medicines. For the purpose of adequately assessing the terrible price the American public is paying for this tragic injustice, let's imagine what would happen if DNP were returned to legal status as a prescription medicine. Overweight people could take a pill and in relative comfort and safety, lose weight in pretty much the same way they would with aerobic exercise: at the rate of around 10 pounds a month. In a few months, there would be very few overweight people left. In a few years, there would be virtually no one left with this problem at all. America would be healthier, happier, more beautiful; a dream come true for countless millions and a financial nightmare for the weight-loss and medical industries.

I have also brought to light and explained who is winning this contest of interests and the sad role manipulation of governmental power plays in this tragedy.

Will this knowledge of these truths lead to the just victory of the American People being given this providentially perfect fat reduction therapy? Or will the few intrepid Americans successfully using DNP, in spite of FDA fiat and caprice, continue to be forced to be **Illegally Thin?**

PART TWO

Clinical Study Reports

"The FDA serves as the pharmaceutical industry's watchdog, which can be called upon to attack and destroy a potential competitor under the guise of protecting the public."

-----James P. Carter, M.D

CHAPTER FIFTEEN

Clinical Report #1
Use of Dinitrophenol in Nutritional Disorders:
A Critical Survey of Clinical Results

The following report is the critical analyses of expert clinical doctors on DNP for human therapeutic use. This report is based on the most extensive series of clinical tests ever done in this country. Doctors Cutting, Stockton and Tainter of Stanford University are the preeminent experts on human therapeutic use of DNP. This report is included here in its entirety so you can see the conclusions of these great clinicians regarding DNP.

Use of Dinitrophenol in Nutritional Disorders:
A Critical Survey of Clinical Results'
By: MAURICE L. TAINTER, M.D., WINDSOR C. CUTTING, M.D., AND B. STOCKTON, M.D.,
Associate Professor of Pharmacology; Resident in Medicine; and Instructor in Therapeutics; Stanford University School of Medicine, San Francisco, Calif.

A LITTLE over a year ago, our first clinical report on dinitrophenol appeared in the Journal of the American Medical Association. Supported in part by grants from the Rockefeller Fluid Research Fund of the School of Medicine, Stanford University, and by Grant from the Committee on Scientific Research of the American Medical Association. Read before the Food and Nutrition Section of the American Public Health Association at the Sixty-third Annual Meeting in Pasadena, Calif., September 3, 1934.

The interest in and enthusiasm for this product were so great that its widespread use has become a matter of some concern in public health. The total amount of the drug being used is astonishing. For instance, during the past year, the Stanford Clinics have supplied to physicians, or to patients on physicians' prescriptions, over 1,200,000 capsules of dinitrophenol of gm. each. Since the usual daily dose is about 3 such capsules and the average duration of treatment about 3 months, this corresponds to 4,500 patients treated with the drug in a year.

In addition, upward of 20 wholesale drug firms are marketing the compound, which suggests that a considerable population is being medicated. Probably at least 100,000 persons have been treated with the drug in this country alone. But this is not all, for reports of its clinical use have also appeared in the medical press of Canada, Great Britain, France, Sweden, Italy, and Australia. Therefore, it appeared timely to summarize the accumulated knowledge of the clinical effects of this drug, and to assess the results critically, in order to determine, if possible, the present status of this new therapeutic agent.

HISTORY

We began to study the actions of alpha dinitrophenol 2-4 first in animals and then in patients, in 1931, being stimulated to do so by the animal experiments of Heymans,[2] who used a similar compound, namely, dinitronaphthol. Dinitrophenol was not new, since it had been known as a dye for about a hundred years, and as an industrial poison for 32 years. There was some interest in its toxicology during the war, due to poisoning in munitions factories. Fundamental investigations of the actions of the compound were made at that time by Magne, Mayer, and collaborators in France, although their studies were not published until 16 years later, i.e., in 1932.

Our experimental results and those of all other investigators are in essential agreement on the remarkable powers of dinitrophenol for augmenting oxidative metabolism by a direct action on the tissues or cells. Prior to our work, there was no indication in any of the published papers that this potent metabolic stimulant might be of any therapeutic usefulness. Therefore, when we first drew attention to the possibility of producing metabolic changes in man with small non-
160

toxic doses of dinitrophenol, there was presented to the medical profession a new tool for use in metabolic disorders.

MEDICAL USES

It has been shown that dinitrophenol can be used to keep the metabolism at an increased level for prolonged periods of time. An increase in the metabolic rate of about 50 per cent can be maintained in most patients without difficulty, by proper selection of dosage; in fact, greater increases have been repeatedly produced. Rabinowitch and Fowler [18] state that they have found difficulty in standardizing the oral dose because of individual variability. Examination of their data shows that, when the probable error of clinical metabolic readings is considered, the agreement is as good as could be expected. Variability in sensitivity to drugs of all kinds is a matter of common knowledge, so that, if perfectly reproducible changes were claimed, it would throw doubt on the validity of the observations. In contrast to Rabinowitch, Dunlop[7] finds a reasonably good agreement between the metabolic stimulation and the size of the dose, which confirms our experience. However, in treating ambulatory patients 6 it is desirable to proceed conservatively by starting with small doses and increasingthem, if necessary, according to the degree of response elicited.

When the drug is taken in adequate dosage, the increased metabolic activity burns extra fat and carbohydrate and thereby reduces body weight.[6] It is very interesting that the protein does not seem to be appreciably affected in the combustion process, as indicated by nitrogen excretion. Accordingly, the tissue framework tends to be conserved. [7, 8, 14] In a preliminary report on the loss of body weight in obese individuals,[6] it was stated that losses of to 3 pounds a week could be obtained with doses of dinitrophenol which were well tolerated. Three other groups of workers have confirmed this result in smaller groups of patients,[7, 9, 10] and it is now a common experience with many practising physicians. Dunlop[7] compared the relative efficiency of thyroid and dinitrophenol in reducing weight in a few selected patients. He found that thyroid upset the water balance of the body in such a way as to cause at once a rapid loss of weight by dehydration. On the other hand, dinitrophenol reduced the weight less rapidly, but in proportion to the metabolic increase and not by an effect on water balance. His experimental results do not satisfactorily establish his conclusion that " even in maximum therapeutic doses it (dinitrophenol) does not compare, as a weight reducer, with thyroid "; since he used both drugs for only a few days at a time, and during these periods the weight changes were so small as to be readily accounted for by shifts in the water balance. The amount of permanent weight change that can be produced by dehydration in non-edematous patients is not great enough to be important where any significant amount of weight is to be lost. If this were not the case, simple dehydration procedures would answer the needs of this difficult clinical problem. Therefore, it appears to us that, before the therapeutic efficiencies of these drugs may be satisfactorily compared, it is necessary to make observations over long periods of time, during which more than a few pounds are lost. It has been indicated by us in several publications [11, 12] that dinitrophenol cannot be used to replace thyroid secretion. It is therefore misleading to compare the intensities of their actions since they act so differently qualitatively.

Since dinitrophenol can increase the tissue metabolism by a direct action on the cells, without producing the sideactions which accompany metabolic stimulation by thyroid, it offers, theoretically at least, interesting possible applications in medicine, besides its use in obesity. For instance, there have been reported interesting effects in psychiatric conditions,[13 14] and failure to relieve myxedema,[7 18] and many other studies are in progress. Because of its widespread and probably sometimes indiscriminate use by large numbers of people, it is pertinent to consider possible harmful effects from the compound.

FATAL EFFECTS

In experimental animals, a large enough dose of dinitrophenol will stimulate the heat production to the point where fatal fever results. The heat production may be increased 1,200 per cent, the body temperature increasing 0.2° C. per minute. Under these conditions, death is caused by heat rigor, that is, by heat-coagulation of tissues. Exactly similar effects can be produced in man provided a large enough dose is taken. This was seen occasionally in munition workers during the World War, who absorbed large amounts of dinitrophenol through the lungs or skin. The first case of fatal poisoning from the therapeutic use of the drug was that of a physician who took a tremendous dose on two separate occasions, with the alleged object of treating an imaginary syphilitic infection.[15] In his second administration, he took 5 gm. of the drug as a single dose, which is a 17 day supply for most patients. A fatal fever resulted, with death in 12 hours.

The second death was a girl who bought the drug on her own responsibility from a druggist. On the fourth day of medication, she took 0.8 gm., which caused a fatal pyrexia.[16] Since the daily dose during the first week or two should be only 0.1 gm.,[6] it is obvious that this girl took a very excessive dose. In fact, it was a larger dose than we have ever used therapeutically, even after months of continuous medication.

The third death occurred in a psychiatric patient who was receiving doses within the therapeutic range.[13] The clinical history of this patient's illness and death is completely at variance with the known actions of dinitrophenol, since there was a protracted course of illness and an absence of serious fever. Also, the autopsy and clinical studies were so incomplete as to preclude a correct diagnosis of the cause of death.

These three cases represent the reported fatalities from dinitrophenol. If the third case be excluded because of the question as to the true cause of the death, it is seen that neither of the other two cases was due to the use of the drug in the usual therapeutic doses. When one considers that some one hundred thousand patients have been treated with this exceedingly potent therapeutic agent, it is a matter of some gratification to know that fatalities have not been more numerous. It might be added in this connection that fatalities from the fever of dinitrophenol can be largely prevented, in animals at least, by chilling the skin with ice packs and by giving oxygen inhalations.[17]

There are also a number of observed, or theoretically possible, deleterious actions, which do not result fatally. These may be discussed according to the organs involved, i.e., skin, liver, kidneys, circulation, and gastrointestinal tract.

SKIN REACTIONS

In a series of 113 obese individuals,[6] we observed the presence of skin rashes in about 7 per cent of cases. The rashes consisted of maculo-papular dermatitis, urticaria, or angio-neuroticlike swellings of the skin, accompanied by pruritus and occasionally by desquamation. There was usually a prodrome of itching before the skin lesions developed.

Four similar cases have been reported to date,[9] [19, 20, 21] and many more than these have undoubtedly occurred. Dintenfass[22] has recorded still another case in which the dermatitis was associated with congestion of the middle ear. The inference might possibly be drawn from certain reports that a Derrien reaction with the urine could be used as a means of predicting possible lack of tolerance to the drug.

This idea rests on a misunderstanding of the nature of the test; it is merely the well-known diazo reaction, which is positive in the presence of amino-nitrophenols. Hence, it only indicates that dinitrophenol has been absorbed in the body and has appeared in the urine in a reduced form. During the war, this reaction was used solely as a means of identifying those workers whose exposure resulted in appreciable absorption of the drug.[23] Bolliger has recently cast doubt on the value of the reaction for even this purpose.[24]

Another possible way of predicting dermal intolerance is by the usual allergic skin tests. Frumess[20] states that, in a case of urticaria, he was able to reproduce the skin-sensitivity by passive transfer. However, an extensive series of skin tests[25] in patients with and without skin rashes, who received dinitrophenol therapeutically, has failed to bring out any evidence that skin sensitivity can be detected by patch, scratch, or intradermal wheal tests. Passive transfer tests were also negative.

These methods would therefore seem unpromising as means of selecting patients for dinitrophenol medication. Since the skin rashes may be very unpleasant or alarming in some cases, they constitute the main disadvantage in the therapeutic use of dinitrophenol. A saving feature, however, is that about half the patients who have had one skin reaction are able, after a short interval, to resume the medication without further difficulty.

LIVER DAMAGE

Much has been made by some editorial writers and clinical reporters of the possibility that dinitrophenol might damage the liver. This has been based mainly on reasoning by analogy from picric acid and other compounds. Since the dinitrophenol has a yellow color, which imparts an icteric tint to the blood plasma, it may be mistaken for the bile pigments of jaundice.[26] The differentiation from the latter may be readily made by adding dilute hydrochloric acid to the plasma which decolorizes the dye. In one patient suspected of liver injury, Rabinowitch " found only a slight increase in the bilirubin in the blood and no change in the urobilinogen. At the next examination of this patient, the findings were all negative. Another case where liver injury was apparently produced has been recently reported by Sidel.[34] We have seen no evidences of damage to the liver in our clinical cases,[6] and at this time we may add more extensive data on this question. In 17 patients who were given an average of 0.3 gm. of sodium dinitrophenol daily for from I to 5 months, there were made 22 determinations of the icteric indices oftheir acidified blood plasmas. The average value was 8. 2 units with a range of from 4.8 to 16.3. Fourteen determinations on non-medicated patients gave an average index of 7.6, with a range of from 4.2 to 10.0. I 45 patients, the bilirubin content of the blood serum was determined by the van den Bergh reaction.* This group of patients received an average daily dose of 0.3 gm. (range 0.1 to 0.6 gm.) for an average period of 19 weeks

165

(range to 50 weeks). The average total amount of the drug taken was 36 gm., with a range of from 2.8 to 122.5 gm.

In these patients, the bilirubin averaged 0.29 units, with a range of from 0. 13 to 0.79 units. Only 2 patients of the 45 showed values over 0.5, but these had no demonstrable clinical evidence of liver disturbance.

If the dinitrophenol injured the liver progressively, it might be expected that the bilirubin of the blood would increase with the total amount of the drug taken. The following tabulation shows that no such increase was present, which further supports the conclusion that damage to the liver was not produced in these patients.

Average total amount of dinitrophenol taken in grams	Number of cases	Bilirubin Units (average)
1-10.0	0	0.27
10.1-30.0	12	0.34
30.1-40.0	8	0.32
40.1-80.0	14	0.22
80.1-122.5	84	0.31

The van den Bergh reaction was repeated in 6 patients some time after stoppage of the dinitrophenol medication. These patients had been off the drug for an average of 36 weeks when they showed an average bilirubin content of 0. 24 units (range 0. 15 to 0. 40). Accordingly, there was no evidence of delayed liver damage.

It has been observed by [15] by Poole and Haining[16] that, in fatal dinitrophenol poisoning, destructive changes may occur in the liver as well as in other viscera. It must be remembered that death in these cases was accompanied by a very high fever, which in itself is enough to account for the morphological changes observed in the liver cells. The usual therapeutic doses of the drug produce no change in body temperature and also no evidences of change in liver function. However, the possibility must still be left open that in occasional patients an idiosyncrasy may exist which might mediate damages to the liver.

KIDNEY

If dinitrophenol in therapeutic doses damaged the kidneys, this would be manifested by albuminuria and related changes. Such evidences could scarcely go undiscovered, since urinalysis is such a common routine procedure. Hence, it becomes of significance that only 1 possible case of renal injury has been reported thus far. Rabinowitch and Fowler [18] reported 1 patient who developed an albuminuria and high blood urea during dinitrophenol medication.

Three weeks later, the urine, and the blood urea and creatinine were all normal. In our patients [6] albuminuria has never been produced by the drug, but on the contrary a limited number of patients have lost their preexisting albuminurias during the medication.

Our experimental studies [27, 30] on animals have also shown the drug to be quite devoid of toxic effects on the kidneys. Therefore, the possibility of renal damage would appear so remote as to cause little or no concern in the therapeutic use of the drug.

CIRCULATION

One of the most striking features of the metabolic stimulation of dinitrophenol is a lack of significant changes in blood pressure or pulse rate, unless therapeutic doses are exceeded." [6] That is, the metabolism may be increased as much as 50 per cent without demonstrable changes in circulatory activity.

This phenomenon is in striking contrast to the effects of thyroid administration, where circulatory changes are a marked feature of the symptom complex.

Confirmation of this early finding has been given by Looney and Hoskins,[14] Rabinowitch,[18] and Dunlop, [7] and more recently again by ourselves working under different conditions. [28] We have observed that, when a patient feels very hot and flushed, there is a rise in venous pressure. This may be the result of vasodilatation in the skin rather than- the metabolic stimulation, since the venous pressure changes do not correlate with those of metabolism. Rosenblum [35] observed inpatients whose metabolic rates were increased 37 per cent by dinitrophenol, that the circulation time from the arm to the tongue was unchanged. This would be in keeping with the lack of changes in the blood pressure and pulse rate previously reported.

Masserman and Goldsmith [13] have made the rather startling claim that 5 out of their 18 psychiatric patients showed toxic effects characterized by a fall of blood pressure, tachycardia, stupor, etc. No such effects were observed by Looney and Hoskins [14] in a similar goup of patients, nor in upward of 300 non-psychotic patients observed by us. Not a single case of hypotension has been observed by, or reported to, us and none has been reported in the literature. The unconfirmed and possibly misinterpreted observations of circulatory changes by Masserman and Goldsmith, taken together with an unexplained death amongtheir patients, suggests that there may have been some error in the therapeutic procedures they used, such as the possible use of a wrong isomer or an impure preparation of dinitrophenol.

Patients who have hypertension can be medicated with dinitrophenol like other patients. As they lose weight, the hypertension is usually improved[6] and the associated symptoms are ameliorated.

BLOOD

In studying the possibility that dinitrophenol might affect the blood, both the red and white corpuscles must be considered. Thus far we have not made extensive red cell counts in patients receiving dinitrophenol, but there have been no evidences of anemia, even after months of medication. The oxygen capacity of the blood of 15 patients was determined for possible evidences of injury to the respiratory function of the blood. Since the normal oxygen capacity of the blood varies from 18 to 21 vols. per cent and in these medicated patients the average value was 19.5 vols. per cent with arange of from 18 to 22 per cent, there is no reason to believe that the blood was injured. These patients received an average of 0.3 gm. sodium dinitrophenol daily, for an average period of 6 weeks. The addition of sodium dinitrophenol, in concentrated solution to several specimens of blood did not change the oxygen capacity. Therefore, the drug does not appear to affect the hemoglobin of the blood in vitro and in vivo.

Study was also made of the fragility of the red cells of these same patients to determine whether there was any increased tendency of the cells to hemolyze. The cells were exposed to various strengths of hypotonic salt solution and the concentrations at which hemolysis began and was complete were noted.[29] Hemolysis of normal cells begins at from 0.46 to 0.38 per cent concentration and is complete at from 0.34 to 0.25 per cent. With the cells of the medicated patients, the hemolysis began at an average of 0.44 per cent, with a range of from 0.42 to 0.46 percent, and was complete at an average of 0.31 per cent, with a range from 0.25 to 0.38 per cent. Since these values were all within the normal range, there was no evidence of alteration in fragility of the red cells.

Current emphasis on the problem of agranulocytosis makes it desirable to observe the white blood cells in patients receiving dinitrophenol. We have seen no cases of malignant neutropenia, or of any condition which might be ascribed to a reduction in the number of white blood cells, among the considerable number of patients treated at Stanford.

In addition, we have examined the blood and bone marrow of dogs given extra-therapeutic doses of dinitrophenol daily for 6 months without finding any abnormalities.[30] However, Hoffman, Butt, and Hickey [31] have reported 1 patient who developed a neutropenia while taking dinitrophenol, and who recovered.

A second case has recently been reported,[36] and other unpublished cases have apparently occurred.[33] Agranulocytosis has been reported in association with medication with a large number of unrelated drugs, and even in the absence of medication. Although the cause of agranulocytosis is not yet understood, it is probable that the underlying factor common to all cases is a defective bone-marrow which require some, and apparently sometimes a relatively insignificant, exciting cause to precipitate the crisis. Given such bonemarrow, it is conceivable that many extraneous agents, physical, bacterial'or chemical, and including even dinitrophenol, might initiate the'clinical syndrome.

The fact is that the vast majority of patients can take massive doses of the various drugs alleged to cause agranulocytosis without damage to white cells, and yet in a sensitive individual even a small therapeutic dose of one of these drugs may suffice to precipitate the condition. However this may be, we shall continue to examine all patients receiving dinitrophenol with the possibility of agranulocytosis in mind, and hope to present more specific data on the question at some future time.

GASTROINTESTINAL TRACT

Heymans has stated that dinitrophenol causes very severe gastroenteritis and loss of appetite, and suggested that the loss of weight was due to the failure or inability of the patient to eat.[32] In our very large series of patients, there have been only 3 cases with digestive complaints during the medication with dinitrophenol.

These complaints lasted only for a few days, such as might be expected from a slight dietary indiscretion. The claim that this drug is a severe irritant to the gastrointestinal tract of patients is unwarranted for doses of therapeutic range, according to our experience and to that of large numbers of physicians prescribing it. Tissues from the gastrointestinal tracts of dogs given the drug for 6 months by mouth also showed no evidences of abnormal changes.[31]

Therefore, there is no good reason for postulating a hypothetical gastroenteritis as the cause of the loss of body weight in the face of repeatedly demonstrated metabolic stimulation, which does adequately account for it.

DISCUSSION AND SUMMARY

It can now be said that dinitrophenol is of definite value as a drug for treating obesity and perhaps some other metabolic disorders. In the hands of the medical profession, it can be used with the maximum benefit and with minimum deleterious results. Unfortunately, its sale cannot be confined to physicians under present legal regulations. As a result, it can be, and is being sold in patent and proprietary medicines under names, which do not reveal its presence. A person buying such an anti-fat remedy over the drugstore counter, with no more directions as to its use, or warning of possible harmful effects, than the manufacturer pleases to put on the label, may run a serious danger of doing himself harm.

This problem is particularly pressing since " obesity cures " are extensively bought by fat people for self-medication without diagnosis. Therefore, it would seem desirable that dinitrophenol be added to the poison list, and its sale regulated so it could not be obtained except on a physician's prescription.

In the first enthusiasm for a new drug, which has spectacular actions, it is to be expected that it may be used somewhat too freely. This we have consistently tried to prevent in the case of dinitrophenol by stressing the potential dangers of the compound when used indiscriminately. Certainly, it should not be used as a routine measure in any clinical condition. Obesity can be controlled in most cases by the physician who will patiently supervise the dietary regime. In other cases, thyroid or thyroxine may be needed. It is only when all other measures have been thoroughly tried and found ineffective, and when there is impelling need for weight reduction, that dinitrophenol medication, with a knowledge of attending risks, should be undertaken. Under these circumstances, the physician must balance the prospective benefit against the potential harm, just as he does with any therapeutic procedure, and give the patient his best chance.

This summary of the clinical effects and side actions of dinitrophenol shows that in some respects this drug is not ideal as a therapeutic agent, since it may cause certain undesired side-actions in a portion of the patients treated. However, this does not mean that it cannot be used safely under proper conditions.

Investigations are under way in our own and many other laboratories to develop new compounds which may be better than this original or parent substance.

It would be only a matter of chance, if dinitrophenol happened to be better than any substitute that could subsequently be prepared. Therefore, it may be expected that the next few years will see other compounds brought forward and advocated. Perhaps some one of them may supplant alpha dinitrophenol as the agent of choice. However, this will in no way affect the great significance of dinitrophenol as having been the first foreign agent, or drug, to be demonstrated as a very potent and well nigh universal metabolic stimulant, which was available for experimental purposes and useful for alleviation of human infirmity.

REFERENCES
1. Cutting, W. C., Mehrtens, H. G., and Tainter, M. L. Actions and Uses of Dinitrophenol. Promising Metabolic Applications. *J.A.M.A.,* 101:193, 1933.
2. Heymans, C., and Bouckaert, J. J. Hyperthermic and Cardiovascular Actions of Dinitro-a-naphthol in the Dog. *Arch. Intern. de Pharm. et de Therap.,* 35:63, 1928.
3. Leymann. Accidents in the Manufacture of Nitrophenol and Nitrochlor-Compounds. *Concordia,* 9:55, 1902.
4. Magne, H., Mayer, A., Plantefol, L. ct al. Studies on the Action of Dinitrophenol 1-2-4 (Thermol). *Ann. de Physiol. et de Physicochem. Biol.,* 8:1-167, 1932.
5. Cutting, W. C., and Tainter, M. L. Actions of Dinitrophenol. *Proc. Soc. Exper. Biol. & Med.,* 29:1268, 1932.
  Tainter, M. L., and Cutting, W. C. Febrile, Respiratorv and Some Other Actions of Dinitrophenol. *J. Pharmacol. & Exper. Therap.,* 48:410, 1933. Miscellaneous Actions of Dinitrophenol. Repeated Administrations, Antidotes, Fatal Doses, Antiseptic Tests and Actions of Some Isomers. Ibid, 49:187.
  Tainter, M. L., Boyes, J. H., and DeEds, F. Actions of Dinitrophenol in Diabetic Dogs. *Arch. Intern. de Pharm. et de Therap.,* 45:235, 1933.
  Hall, V. E., Field, J., Sahyun, M., Cutting, W. C., and Tainter, M. L. Carbohydrate Metabolism, Respiration and Circulation in Animals with Basal Metabolism Heightened by Dinitrophenol. *Am. J. Physiol.,* 106:432, 1933.
  Emge, L. A., Wulff, L. M. R., and Tainter, M. L. Effects of Dinitrophenol on an Experimental Sarcoma of the White Rat. *Proc. Soc. Exper. Biol. & Med.,* 31:152, 1933.
  Tainter, M. L. Dinitrophenol in Diet, on Growth and Duration of Life of the White Rat. Proc. Soc. Exper. Biol. & Med., 31:1161, 1934.

6. Tainter, M. L., Stockton, A. B., and Cutting, W. C. Use of Dinitrophenol in Obesity and Related Coniditions. A Progress Report. *J.A.M.A.*, 101:1472, 1933.

7. Dunlop, D. M. The Use of 2-4 Dinitrophenol as a Metabolic Stimulant. *Brit. M. J.*, 3820:524, 1934.

8. Cutting, W. C., and Tainter, M. L. Metabolic Actions of Dinitrophenol with the Use of Balanced and Unbalanced Diets. *J.A.M.A.*, 101 :2p99, 1933.

9. Anderson, H. H., Reed, A. C., and Emerson, G. A. Toxicity of Alpha-Dinitrophrenol. Report of a Case. *J.A.M.A.*, 101:1053, 1933.

10. Courdouan. Nitrophenine: An Accelerator of Cellular Oxidation. *Progrps Med.*, 41:1738, 1933.

11. Cutting, C. C., and Tainter, M. L. Comparative Effects of Dinitrophenol and Thyroxin on Tadpole Metamorphosis. *Proc. Soc. Exper. Biol. & Med.*, 31:97, 1933.

12. Cutting, W. C., Rytand, D., and Tainter, M. L. Relationship Between Blood Cholesterol and Increased Metabolism from Dinitrophenol and Thyroid. *J. Cliiv. Investigation*, 13:547, 1934.

13. Masserman, J. H., and Goldsmith, H. Dinitrophenol: Its Therapeutic and Toxic Actions in Certain Types of Psychobiologic Underactivity. *J.A.M.A.*, 102:523, 1934.

14. Looney, J. M., and Hoskins, R. G. The Effect of Dinitrophenol on the Metabolism as Seen in Schizophrenic Patients. *New Eng. J. Med., 210: 1206, 1934.*

15. Tainter, Al. L., and Wood, D. A. A Case of Fatal Dinitrophenol Poisoning. *J.A.M.A.*, 102:1147,1934.

16. Poole, F. E., and Haining, R. B. Sudden Death from Dinitrophenol Poisoning. Report of a Case with Autopsy. *J.A.M.A.*, 102:1141, 1934.

17. Tainter, M. L. Low Oxygen Tensions and Temperatures on the Actions and Toxicity of Dinitrophenol. *J. Pharm. Exper. Therap.*, 51:45, 1934.

18. Rabinowitch, I. M., and Fowler, A. F. Dinitrophenol. *Canad. M. A. J.*, 30:128, 1934.

19. Hirsch, S. Report of a Toxic Manifestation Due to " Dinitrenal." *J.A.M.A.*, 102:950, 1934.

20. Frumess, G. M. Allergic Reaction to Dinitrophenol. Report of a Case. *J.A.M.A.*, 102:1219, 1934.

21. Jackson, H., and Duvall, A. I. Dinitrophenol Poisoning. Report of a Case. *J.A.M.A.,* 102:1844, 1934.

22. Dintenfass, H. An Ear Complication from Dinitrophenol Medication. *J.A.M.A.*, 102:838, 1934.

23. Guerbet. *L'Expertise Chimique Dans Les Cas D'Intoxication Par le Dinitrophenol,* 1918. Ministere de l'Armement et des Fabrications de Guerre. Conference Pour l'Etude de la Toxicite des Explosifs (Paris).

24. Bolliger, A. Detection and Estimation of a-Dinitrophenol, New Drug for the Treatment of Obesity. *M. J. Australia*, 1:367, 1934.

25. Matzger, E. Can Sensitivity to Dinitrophenol be Determined by Skin Tests? *J.A.M.A.*, 103:253,1934.

26. Haft, H. H. Toxicity of Dinitrophenol. *J.A.M.A.*, 101:1171, 1933.

27. Schulte, T. L., and Tainter, M. L. Chronic Toxicity of Dinitrophenol: Renal Function. *Proc. Soc. Exper. Biol. & Med.,* 31:1163, 1934.

28. Stockton, A. B., and Cutting, W. C. Clinical Circulatory Effects of Dinitrophenol. *J.A.M.A.* In press.

29. Todd, J. C., and Sanford, A. H. *Clinical Diagnosis by Laboratory Methods,* 1928. 6th ed., p. 363.

30. Tainter, M. L., Cutting, W. C., Wood, D. A., and Proescher, F. *Arch. Path.* In press.

31. Hoffman, A. M., Butt, E. M., and Hickey, N. G. Neutropenia Following Amidopyrine: Preliminary Report. *J.A.M.A.*, 102:1213, 1934.

32. Heymans, C. The Influence of Some New Nitroderivatives on the Cellular Metabolism and on Body Temperature. *J. Pharm. Exper. Therap.*, 51: 144, 1934.

33. Kracke, R. R. Personal Communication.

34. Sidel, N. Dinitrophenol Poisoning Causing Jaundice: Report of a Case. *J.A.M.A.*, 103:254, 1934.

35. Rosenblum, H. *The Rate of Blood Flow in Patients Receiving Dinitrophenol.* In press.

36. Bohn, S. S. Agranulocytic Angina Following Ingestion of Dinitrophenol. J.A.M.A. 103:249 1934.

CHAPTER SIXTEEN

Clinical Report #2
Patent Document for DNP

Human weight loss inducing method

United States Patent 4673691

Abstract:

A human weight reduction method in which 2,4-dinitrophenol and a thyroid hormone preparation are administered to the patient. The dinitrophenol is administered in dosages sufficient to elevate the patient's body temperature, typically 250 mg every other day. The thyroid hormone preparation preferably contains 3,5,3'-triiodothyronine and is administered in dosages sufficient to substantially maintain the patient's serum T3 concentration originally present at treatment onset.

Bachynsky, Nicholas (1110 Pine Cir., Sea Brook, TX, 77586)
Application Number:06/668501
Publication Date:06/16/1987
Filing Date:11/05/1984
Assignee:Bachynsky, Nicholas (Sea Brook, TX)
Primary Class:514/567
Other Classes:514/909
International Classes:*A61K31/06*; *A61K31/195*; **A61K31/045**; **A61K31/185**; A61K31/195
Field of Search:514/728, 514/909, 514/567

US Patent References:

4087554 Method for improving growth rate and feed efficiency May, 1978 Haydock et al. 514/728

Other References:
Chem. Abst. 66:82758c (1967)--Rossini et al.
Chem. Abst. 71:27671x (1969)--Tomita et al.
Chem. Abst. 77:109780v (1972)--Tiller et al.
Chem. Abst. 82:25791q (1975)--Wahl et al.
Chem. Abst. 88:167300b (1978)--Kaplan et al.
Chem. Abst. 89:191455x (1978)--Organesyan et al.
Chem. Abst. 100:168805y (1984)--Sydykov.
Chem. Abst. 102:56608w (1985)--Langer.
Simkins, S., "Dinitrophenol and Desiccated Thyroid in the Treatment of Obesity,"
JAMA 108, pp. 2110-2117 and 2193-2199 (1937).
Tainter, M. L. et al., "Dinitrophenol in the Treatment of Obesity,"

Primary Examiner:Robinson, Douglas W.
Attorney, Agent or Firm:Pravel, Gambrell, Hewitt & Kimball

Claims:

I claim:

1. A method of inducing weight loss in a patient, comprising the steps of:

(a) administering 2,4-dinitrophenol or salt thereof at a rate ranging from about 60 to about 250 mg/day; and

(b) concurrently administering 3,5,3'-triiodothyronine to the patient at a rate ranging from about 25 to about 100 mcg/day.

2. The method of claim 1, wherein said 3,5,3'-triiodothyronine is substantially free of thyroxine.

3. The method of claim 1, wherein said 3,5,3'-triiodothyronine administration is at a rate ranging from about 50 to about 100 mcg/day.

4. The method of claim 1, wherein said dinitrophenol is administered at said rate with dosages given only on alternate days.

5. The method of claim 1, wherein said dinitrophenol is administered at said rate with primary dosages given on alternate days and smaller, supplemental dosages given on the days immediately subsequent to said alternate days.

6. The method of claim 1, wherein 2,4-dinitrophenol is administered.

7. A method of inducing weight loss in a patient, comprising the steps of:

> (a) administering 2,4-dinitrophenol to the patient at a rate ranging from about 125 to about 250 mg/day; and

> (b) concurrently administering 3,5,3'-triiodothyronine substantially free of thyroxine to the patient at a rate ranging from about 50 to about 100 mcg/day.

8. The method of claim 7, wherein said dinitrophenol and said 3,5,3'-triiodothyronine are administered at initial rates of about 250 mg of said dinitrophenol every other day and about 50 mcg 3,5,3'-triiodothyronine per day, and following 2-12 weeks of said

177

administration at said initial rates, are administered at subsequent rates of about 250 mg of said dinitrophenol every other day alternated with about 125 mg of said dinitrophenol on subsequent days and about 100 mcg 3,5,3'-triiodothyronine per day.

Description:

This invention relates to a method of inducing weight loss in patients by the concurrent administration of 2,4-dinitrophenol and 3,5,3'-triiodothyronine.

BACKGROUND OF THE INVENTION

Obesity is a common problem. Simply stated, obesity is an excess accumulation of adipose tissue, which contains fat stored in the form of triglycerides. The number of cells in the body is determined at least by late adolescence and while the number of adipocyte cells may increase, it does not decrease. Thus, weight gain can result from an enlargement of adipocyte cells or an increase in their number. Typically, obese individuals have hypertrophic cells and the severely obese have an increase in adipose cell number as well as hypertrophy. An obese patient only reduces the fat in his cells when he loses weight. Further, he may not ever lose the tendency to gain weight.

Body weight is regulated by an endogenous body mechanism. Physiological and neurological properties establish and maintain a given weight. Briefly stated, glycerol, which is released during hydrolysis of triglycerides and adipose tissue, is widely believed to regulate caloric intake and metabolism. Others have postulated that caloric intake is affected by both body temperature and environmental temperature. In addition, cell size and number affect energy regulation. Weight gain cannot be predicted solely on the amount of calories ingested.

In normal persons, thermogenesis is an adaptive mechanism which increases the metabolic rate after overeating. While a normal person will experience an increase in thermogenesis following increased caloric intake, the obese either has a substantially decreased thermogenic mechanism or lacks this particular mechanism entirely.

178

The use of dinitrophenol to treat obesity is known. Dinitrophenol is known to elevate the body temperature and produces a marked increase in caloric metabolism. However, ingestion of massive amounts of dinitrophenol causes toxicity by the uncoupling of oxidative phosphorylation in the mitochondria of cells. Because of this toxicity, excessive amounts can result in profuse diaphoresis, fever, thirst, tachycardia and respiratory distress which can lead to hyperpyrexia, profound weight loss, respiratory failure and death. The minimum fatal human oral dose is estimated at one to three grams (approximately 20-30 mg/kg).

In methods heretofore known to using dinitrophenol to induce weight loss, while initial daily dosages have usually been much less than the toxic amount, about 100-250 mg, as the treatment progressed the patient normally developed a tolerance for dinitrophenol and the dosage was increased to obtain the same results. This increased dosage led to an increased frequency of toxic symptoms and general disuse of dinitrophenol in inducing weight loss.

It has also been known to use drugs with thyroid hormone activity for the treatment of obesity. However, as described in Physicians' Desk Reference, Medical Economics Co. Inc., (Oradell, N.J.), 37th Ed. (1983), in euthyroid patients, it is well established that doses within the daily hormonal requirements are ineffective for weight reduction. However, larger doses may produce serious or even life-threatening manifestations of toxicity.

SUMMARY OF THE INVENTION

The present invention avoids the necessity of increased dosages of dinitrophenol and the concomitant toxicity problems associated therewith as treatment progresses while obtaining improved results. It has been discovered that the use of dinitrophenol induces hypothyroidism which can be prevented by concurrently administering thyroid hormone preparation with the dinitrophenol.

Briefly, the present invention is a method of inducing weight loss in patients, including the steps of administering dinitrophenol to the patient in an amount sufficient to clinically increase thermogenesis of the patient, and concurrently administering a thyroid hormone

179

preparation to the patient in an amount sufficient to substantially maintain the serum concentration of 3,5,3'-triiodothyronine of the patient originally present at treatment onset.

DETAILED DESCRIPTION OF THE PREFERRED EMBODIMENT

It has been discovered that the ingestion of dinitrophenol induces hypothyroidism. Athough it is not fully understood, it is believed that the normal thyroid gland produces both thyroxine (referred to herein as T4) and 3,5,3'-triiodothyronine (referred to herein as T3). However, approximately eighty percent of the serum T3 present in the body is produced by the extrathyroidal monodeiodination of T4 to T3. When dosages of dinitrophenol are taken, hypothyroidism is induced, not by a reduction in activity of the thyroid, but by a reduction of the rate of extrathyroidal conversion of T4 to T3. While both T4 and T3 are biologically active, T3 is much more active than T4. Thus, the reduction in serum T3 concentration induced by taking dinitrophenol substantially offsets the metabolic effect of the dinitrophenol. By analogy, the reduction in serum T3 concentration is similar to that observed in fasting patients. Typically, normal serum T3 concentration ranges from about 70 to about 200 ng/dl.

It has further been discovered that deficient serum T3 concentrations resulting from administration of dinitrophenol can be restored to normal concentrations by concurrently administering a thyroid hormone preparation therewith.

In practicing the method of this invention, dinitrophenol is administered to the patient. The metabolically active dinitrophenols suitable for use in the invention include 2,4-dinitrophenol and the salts thereof. By the term administration is meant any suitable manner of introducing the medication into the patient's body, including orally (p.o.) and topically. The preferred manner of administering dinitrophenol is orally, as in the form of a tablet or capsule.

The amount of dinitrophenol given should be sufficient so that the patient experiences increased body temperature. Preferably, the body temperature is elevated approximately 1° F. The dose of dinitrophenol required to obtain this result varies from patient to

180

patient, depending on factors such as, for example, weight, age, health, environmental conditions, physical activity, nutrition, and psychological state, but will normally be in the range of from about 60 to about 500 mg per day, or about 0.60 to about 5.0 mg/kg of body weight per day. Preferably, the dinitrophenol is administered in daily or alternating daily dosages, insuring that no cumulative effective results, such as excessive thermogenesis.

It is essential that the amount of dinitrophenol administered not exceed toxic doses. In a few patients, adverse reactions may occur at dosages of dinitrophenol which are not effective to elevate the body temperature, contraindications including any clinical state in which there is hypermetabolism, such as hyperthyroidism, ongoing infections, and pregnancy, and any other clinical conditions such as heart disease, chronic obstructive pulmonary disease, Addison's disease, liver disorders, or renal failure. Most are safely treated with suitable results from the aforementioned dosages.

Concurrently with the administering of the dinitrophenol, or shortly thereafter, a thyroid hormone preparation is administered to the patient. As used herein, the term thyroid hormone preparation includes any suitable preparation which restores the serum T3 concentration, including preparations containing 3,5,3'-triiodothyronine, thyroxine, derivatives thereof or combinations thereof. Preferably, the thyroid hormone preparation contains T3. Because of the varying potency of such preparations, dosages of thyroid harmone preparation are reported herein on a T3 equivalent basis.

The thyroid hormone preparation is administered in an amount sufficient to maintain the pretreatment serum T3 concentration in the patient, typically about 70-200 ng/dl in normal patients. Generally, from about 25 to about 200 mcg T3 equivalent per day, or from about 0.3 to about 2.7 mcg T3 equivalent per kilogram of body weight per day, is sufficient. Preferably, the thyroid hormone preparation is administered daily. In an especially preferred embodiment, the thyroid hormone preparation is administered orally with the dinitrophenol.

As described above, the rate of extrathyroidal conversion of T4 to T3 may vary as treatment with the dinitrophenol progresses. Thus, it may be necessary to increase or decrease the dosage of the thyroid hormone preparation accordingly.

It is preferred that in the practice of the method of this invention, the patient be closely monitored, especially in the initial stages of treatment. Recommended pretreatment and initial treatment protocol includes physical examination, electrocardiogram, and stress electrocardiogram if indicated, complete blood count, urinalysis, thyroid function studies (T3, T4 and reverse T3), serum electrolytes, HDL cholesterol, serum creatinine, blood urea nitrogen, uric acid, calcium, pulmonary function tests and liver function tests including liver enzymes, biliribin, and alkaline phosphatase.

In an especially preferred embodiment, the patient is started on initially lower dosage rates of dinitrophenol, about 250 mg every other day, and thyroid hormone preparation, about 25-50 mcg/day on a T3 equivalent basis. After 2-12 weeks of this treatment, if no adverse reactions are noted, the dosage rates may be increased to about 250 mg dinitrophenol alternated daily with about 125 mg, i.e. 250 mg on even-numbered days and 125 mg on odd-numbered days, and to about 100 mcg/day thyroid hormone preparation on a T3 equivalent basis. When the weight goal of the patient is achieved, the administration of the dinitrophenol may be discontinued, and the thyroid hormone preparation continued to maintain the patient's weight. While dietary control need not be strict, weight loss and weight maintenance are facilitated by moderate caloric intake of less than about 1800 calories per day, during and following treatment.

This method is illustrated by way of the case histories which follow.

Case 1

A white female 31 years of age with a weight in excess of 200 pounds had attempted to loss weight with various diet plans. She had only been able to achieve about a 20-pound loss, and had immediately regained the weight. The patient was nulliparous and had no ongoing medical problems. Upon physical examination, she had a weight of 208.5 pounds, a height of 5 feet, 3 inches, and a blood pressure of 132/80, without any goiter. Laboratory analyses, including complete blood count, liver profile, serum electrolytes, kidney function tests and

182

thyroid function tests, were all within normal limits. Because of her familial history of heart disease, she underwent a stress electrocardiogram which was normal other than early fatigue and calf cramping.

The patient was started on CYTOMEL brand of liothyronine sodium (manufactured by Smith, Kline and French), 50 mcg/day p.o., and on 2,4-dinitrophenol, 250 mg every other day p.o. On the 19th day of medication, the patient had normal vital signs and the dosages were increased to 100 mcg/day liothyronine, and 250 mg/day dinitrophenol alternated every other day with 125 mg/day. The patient was subsequently maintained on these dosages and returned for follow-up examinations approximately every 3 weeks. The weight loss history is seen in Table 1. After 241 days of medication, the patient has achieved her weight goal of 135 pounds. Administration of the dinitrophenol was discontinued and the patient was maintained on liothyronine, 100 mcg/day p.o. No weight gain was subsequently observed.

TABLE 1

Day	Weight (lbs)
1	208 1/2
19	202 1/2
35	196 1/2
49	189 1/2
69	184
92	175
113	167
134	160
155	152 1/2
180	148
206	146
241	135

Case 2

A male 40 years of age with a weight of approximately 250 pounds had attempted to lose weight with a variety of diet plans and diet medications. Success had been limited to 5-10 pound weight losses, with immediate regain. On physical examination, the patient has a height of 5 feet, 10 inches, a weight of 255 pounds and a blood pressure of 160/100. Complete blood count, SMAC, serum electrolytes, thyroid function tests, glucose tolerance tests and stress electrocardiogram were normal.

The patient was started on liothyronine, 50 mcg/day p.o., and on dinitrophenol, 250 mg every other day p.o. After two weeks, the blood pressure returned to normal (130/80), and the dosages were increased to 100 mcg/day liothyronine and 250 mg dinitrophenol alternated daily with 125 mg. The weight loss history is presented in Table 2. Once the weight goal of 167 pounds had been achieved, the patient was taken off the dinitrophenol administration and the 100 mcg/day liothyronine medication was maintained. The patient was instructed to restrict caloric intake to approximately 1800 calories per day. No subsequent weight gain was observed.

TABLE 2

Day	Weight (lbs)
1	255
14	241
30	232
44	227
65	220
76	214
97	208
125	203
153	197 3/4
181	193
209	189
279	178
321	167

Case 3

A white male 38 years of age with a weight of approximately 342 pounds had made numerous attempts to lose weight "with all methods" without any success. Upon physical examination, the patient had a weight of 352 pounds, a height of 5 feet, 11 inches and a blood pressure of 150/110. Other than a slight enlargement of the heart on X-ray and +3 pitting edema, the physical examination was unremarkable. Laboratory analysis initially revealed a blood sugar of 372 with a glycohemoglobin of 14.3 (normal 4.4-8.2). The remaining tests, including stress electrocardiogram, were within normal limits. The patient was started on liothyronine, 50 mcg/day p.o., and dinitrophenol, 250 mg every other day, and was instructed to restrict his caloric intake to approximately 1800 calories per day. On the 59th day of treatment, the dosages were increased to 100 mcg/day liothyronine, and 250 mg/day dinitrophenol alternated every day with 125 mg. The patient's weight loss history is presented in Table 3. Following treatment, the dinitrophenol administration was discontinued and the patient was maintained on liothyronine, 100 mcg/day p.o. and instructed to maintain his caloric intake to approximately 1800 calories per day. No subsequent weight gain was observed.

TABLE 3

Day	Weight (lbs)
1	354
24	333
38	314
59	317
80	297 1/4
101	288
122	275
143	260 1/2
164	254
185	243 1/2
206	246

227	235 1/2
248	234
269	229
290	222

The above cases illustrate the effectiveness of the method with obese patients unable to reduced their weight by conventional methods.

Having described any weight loss method above, many variations in the details thereof will occur to those skilled in the art. It is intended that all such variations which fall within the scope and spirit of the appended claims be embraced thereby.

PART THREE

Modern Day Use and Protocols

**It is dangerous to be right when
the government is wrong.
~Voltaire**

CHAPTER SEVENTEEN

A Few Words About Body Builders

Through my research, I have come to a better understanding of the bodybuilding and fitness community. I have actually gained considerable respect for bodybuilders and their sport through my research of their forums. As a group, I find bodybuilders to be intelligent, informed, passionate, disciplined and dedicated people. Like much of our culture, they can be prone to rough language though.

I think bodybuilders are often misunderstood and get a bad rap in the court of public opinion. Just think about it, bodybuilders are often seen by the public and portrayed by the media as steroid abusers, aggressive, temperamental, indifferent to the law, indulging in unhealthy and dangerous consumption of hormones and chemicals, etc. These public perceptions are as unfortunate, as they are inaccurate.

Take the "unhealthy" epithet for instance. Your average recreational or amateur bodybuilder is in fantastic physical condition. Contrast this with the average American you see in public and there is no comparison. And as far as their health is concerned, as distinct from their physical condition, regarding their hormone and chemical use; the great majority of these guys are incredibly knowledgeable about their bodies and the effects of the substances they use on themselves. There are certainly side effects they have to deal with but they are passionate about their safety and health and are very effective maintaining both, in a very scientific way.

They are also passionate about other body builders being responsible, especially beginners. They lecture these neophytes on the steroid boards about educating themselves and safely and properly doing everything from steroid use to diet and exercise. This passion for safely and properly employing the tools of their sport is manifested in nearly every post on the body building forums. Passion is almost an understatement these guys are adamantly dogmatic and even emotional in their impatience with abusive, foolish and unsafe practices in their sport. The thing that gets them the most upset is when anyone under twenty-five years old attempts to use steroids.

I am not saying that there are not those who indulge in irresponsible and excessive practices in the bodybuilding world. There are, of course, but the community, as a whole does not tolerate the practices of this small group.

I will be covering this subject more extensively in the companion book to this one that is not yet completed. It will cover several other substances that are not allowed by the FDA for fat reduction. Two in particular have absolutely incredible benefits in addition to their fat reduction properties. But, they do not compare to DNP for shear efficacy at fat reduction.

CHAPTER EIGHTEEN

Dosing

Popular Dosing and Cycling Protocols

Before getting to the details of DNP usage, it is important to point out two things. While all clinical studies and known history of use show that DNP is an extremely benign substance, in terms of its direct effect on the body, it does have dose dependent side effects that need to be understood to safely and properly use it. This is true of virtually any drug, medicine, antidote etc.

First, and most obviously, DNP like any ingestible substance can be overdosed to the point of being health threatening or even deadly. DNP shares this attribute with virtually every substance, including water. Water can be deadly, if you drink too much of it, too fast. I am not speaking of drowning, I am saying you can overdose on water and there are cases of it happening, this is called water intoxication.

While DNP does no known direct or serious harm to the body, it does have side effects. The good thing is that these side effects are, for the most part, the same ones that come with the fat burning process that happens during aerobic exercise, for example: overheating, dehydration, exhaustion etc.

A good way to conceptualize the cause of almost all of the side effects of DNP is to realize that they are the result of heat caused by fat burning; not some direct chemical action on the body. DNP is not hurting the user's body, rather through a very basic process it is causing the body to burn fat so efficiently that heat is produced, just like when a person exercises. The difference is that the heat can be

191

> "the fat burning induced heat can be kept at a safe and tolerable level"

raised much higher with DNP than it can be with exercise. A person cannot exercise long enough or with sufficient intensity to cause the same degree of fat burning induced heat that extremely high doses of DNP can cause. This is good news for two reasons. DNP always works its fat burning magic with unstoppable efficiency and the greater the dose, the greater the fat burning; so DNP can burn fat at a higher rate than anything else known. The other good thing is that since DNP's fat burning effect is dose dependent, the fat burning induced heat can be kept at a safe and tolerable level. Another plus is that even at very safe and tolerable heat levels DNP still burns fat off the user's body faster than any other known drug or chemical.

So keep in mind as you read the side effects listed below that they are, for the most part, exactly the same heat related ones that are caused by exercise and become a problem only if you are overdosing or are not taking other common sense precautions you would take when exercising.

All that being said, since overdosing DNP can be a serious issue, I am of the opinion that DNP should be used at the lower level dosing, well below what is considered safe by many modern day users. In other words, dosing should be kept well within the safe and comfortable level. A person can still burn fat faster than with diet and exercise or using other fat reducing substances, it just takes a little longer than at higher doses.

Two forms of DNP

DNP is available in two forms: crystalline (DRY) and raw powder (usually 10-15 percent water). Dry DNP is more efficient mg. for mg. Some DNP "experts" claim that crystalline is almost twice as effective. I have not been able to personally test or verify this, so if a person were to use the raw powder they would need to be aware that they may need to increase the dosages, as the dosing protocols below refer to crystalline DNP. The reason I have used crystalline as the standard is because it is the stronger of the two and so the lower dosed of the two. I figure it's better for people who aren't aware of the difference, to use too little rather than too much.

An often-quoted rule of thumb, by many modern day users for DNP dosing, is 2-6 mg per kg of body weight per day. In my personal experience, 2mg per kg to 5mg per kg per day dosing is very effective. Doses at the lower range, 100-200 mg a day, come with virtually no side effects except an occasional feeling of being a little warm and maybe slightly sweaty or drained. This seems to be the consensus among the few that have actually dosed so low. At 300 to 500 mg per day, the heat is much more pronounced and the side effects of that heat become more of an issue, but still very manageable. At 600mg per day people start to get hot, exhausted and really sweaty. Staying properly hydrated starts to become much more of an issue at this level. Also, various supplements become more important to counteract the heat related issues.

This quote from one study gives a more detailed and professional description:

> *"The amount of dinitrophenol given should be sufficient so that the patient experiences increased body temperature. Preferably, the body temperature is elevated approximately 1.degree. F. The dose of dinitrophenol required to obtain this result varies from patient to patient, depending on factors such as, for example, weight, age, health, environmental conditions, physical activity, nutrition, and psychological state, but will normally be in the range of from about 60 to about 500 mg per day, or about 0.60 to about 5.0 mg/kg of body weight per day. Preferably, the dinitrophenol is administered in daily or alternating daily dosages, insuring that no cumulative effective results, such as excessive thermogenesis."*

There is another dose related issue that should be mentioned here. According to various experts, doses of 200mg a day or less do not shut down the body's conversion of t4 to t3. This is beneficial in a number of ways. These same experts also state, that when this process is shut down due to higher dosing, cycles should be kept shorter.

Thirty days seems to be the higher end of consensus for these heavier dose runs. Many also say, that after discontinuing DNP, the t4 to t3 process returns to normal very quickly. Longer DNP cycles at lower doses seem to have all of the advantages with the obvious exception, that higher doses remove fat quicker. This is the dosing protocol in most of clinical studies I have seen. Generally, they are in the 200mg - 300mg a day range and run over many months with excellent results, usually in the ten pound a month range, and no harmful side effects are reported.

CHAPTER NINETEEN

Side Effects

Please, keep in mind while reading this that the following side effects are dose dependant. At the smaller dosing of 200mg a day or less, these side effects will be minimal or unnoticeable depending on the individual and the conditions in which DNP is used. Conversely, the side effects will be more pronounced as doses are increased.

Also, it is very important to keep in mind is that DNP related side effects are mostly the same side effects observed during exercise. The only difference is that the effects are spread out over a much longer period. If you think about it, as you read the following side effects are a result of this fat burning caused heat, exactly the same as with exercise.

So as long as a person keeps to the lower dosing protocols and takes the same common sense measures he or she would take while exercising, he or she should rarely notice any of these side effects.

I will describe these "sides" as body builders, who use high doses of DNP describe them. Some of these guys use very high doses, putting themselves through a lot of inconvenience and discomfort to achieve their high-speed fat loss goals. Their experiences will illustrate specifically why lower dosing protocols are to be preferred from a mere comfort and convenience standpoint, not to mention safety.

All of these side effects, with the exception of water retention, will subside 24-48 hours after discontinuing use of DNP.

Heat and Overheating

At 600mg of DNP a day or above, the heat generated can become quite annoying and inconvenient. The body's temperature only goes up one or two degrees because the heat is radiated away from the body. DNP is not really raising the body's temperature. It is causing fat burning, that is producing heat. Even this fat burning is not a process that directly increases body temperature or anything like that. It is more like getting warm by standing next to a fire or heater. Even though the heat is being radiated off and out, it is still a heat source affecting everything around it. At higher doses a person on DNP can put off enough heat, that someone sitting next to them can feel it.

Your body uses the same vasodilatation, sweating etc. to help this heat dispersing process on DNP, that it does when a person is jogging. A person should take the same precautions one would for aerobic exercise. For example, it is not good to do extensive running in 100 degree plus weather and it is not good to use DNP in those conditions either. The body will not be able to throw off the heat effectively when the ambient temperature is so high. During DNP use, a person should try to stay indoors with air conditioning. At low doses a person will have a lot more latitude with what he or she can comfortably get away with. This of course will vary a little with the individual. Everyone is different. Use common sense. For instance, I know of a case where a man taking 450 mg of DNP a day went into a 200 degree sauna. There is no way for your body to properly radiate off the heat, when the ambient temperature is greater than your body temperature. He came out of it ok, but I am glad I found out about it, so I could point out the risks involved, in this book.

Dehydration

While fat-burning produced heat is the underlying cause of DNP related side effects, dehydration is perhaps the one that is of greatest concern. This is because it is hard to tell how dehydrated a person is becoming, while on DNP. Somehow DNP seems to mask dehydration and thirst. A person just doesn't feel as thirsty as he or she really is. For this reason, body builders and others that use high doses stress the risk of dehydration more than any other risk. At higher doses the dangers of dehydration are very real and not to be taken lightly.

These high dose users often drink two or three gallons of water a day to stay hydrated. Another way to keep dehydration down is to take a combination of pyruvate and glycerine. This will be covered more in the supplements section.

At lower doses, it is still important to drink more water than usual, because even though one may not feel like it, he or she will be a little more dehydrated than usual. Most people don't drink enough water anyway and are chronically dehydrated. Before beginning DNP use, a person should make sure that he or she is truly hydrated by consuming proper amounts of water for several days. Studies show that a gallon of water can be consumed per day by an adult for proper hydration.

Lethargy

While the two above-mentioned side effects are of greatest concern, feeling tired and drained is probably the most annoying. Being on DNP is like a long slow jog all day long in terms of energy depletion because the same thing is happening as with jogging, the body's ATP is being depleted. At lower doses it will be barely noticeable, unless the person is exerting himself. At high doses, it can be quite intense, depending on the individual. Everything becomes tiring and some of these high dose users end up lying around feeling exhausted. Remember, this is not because DNP is injuring them in some way, it is because DNP use has caused them to be drained of energy like exercising does. Some clinicians specifically make note of this fact. There are various ways for a person to combat this tired feeling:

- ❖ Stay on lower doses of DNP

- ❖ Don't exercise or unnecessarily exert the body

- ❖ Eat high carbohydrate foods, especially fruit.

- ❖ Take supplements (listed in the supplement section below).

Sweating

Sweating is a side effect that is more of a problem for some people, than it is for others. For instance, this is something that I did not have a problem with. I don't really sweat much anyway, so that and the fact that it was winter are probably the reasons I did not have this problem. Obviously, sweating is fat burning heat related. This is also the reason people sweat when exercising.

The best solutions are just the same ones you would use when working out:

- ❖ Wear lighter clothing than normal whenever possible

- ❖ Keep the air conditioning on if necessary and when possible

- ❖ At night a fan can help a lot

- ❖ Lower dosing is always a solution, if the sweat is overly bothersome

Water retention

Water retention seems to affect all users, but it is also dose dependent, as with all DNP sides. This is really not a problem for anyone, as far as I can tell from all of my studies of clinical and private use. Just keep in mind, that while a person is on DNP, he or she will not see the full benefits of the fat loss until 3-7 days after discontinuing the use. DNP water retention always clears in this time frame. While there is not much a person can do about the water retention, at least that I can find in my research, there is something that a person should absolutely never ever do while on DNP, and that is to take any kind of diuretic. While on DNP, the body is already having to fight dehydration, and diuretics will exacerbate that condition considerably. At higher DNP dosing it is generally considered dangerous to take a diuretic. Also most diuretics are not very effective because they operate on the anti diuretic hormone (ADH) and DNP water retention is independent of ADH. A person should not use diuretics in the week after DNP use, while the water is clearing from his or her system, as it can accelerate electrolyte depletion and that is not good either. The body's electrolytes will already be depleted because of sweating. Drinking V8® juice is considered one of the best solutions.

Shortness of breath or rapid breathing.

A slightly elevated or labored breathing is normal as it is part of the body's reaction to increased metabolism, like when a person exercises.

This symptom is more pronounced at higher doses of DNP. It is the opinion of many users, including myself, that, if it is very pronounced at all, this is a strong indicator that your dose is simply too high. Most recommend discontinuing use until breathing becomes normal and restart with lower the doses. Makes sense to me.

Nausea

Nausea is another possible side effect of DNP. It does not seem to be chronic, but can just pop up. Perhaps, this is from being dehydrated. This is the only side effect, besides feeling a little warm, that I had at 400mg a day. I got it early on and only once. It happened right after a large dinner of spicy Mexican food and lasted about an hour.

Rash Allergy

According to available clinical statistics, about 7% of DNP users will get a rash. A rash often starts with no other symptom other than itching. It will later develop into a rash that can spread to almost anywhere on the skin. It seems that it is not too big of an issue as it is alleviated with an over the counter antihistamine. There is another method used to cure the rash if it develops. It seems that a tolerance is built up with DNP related allergic reactions over time and repeated use. When a person notices the rash, he or she discontinues use for 5 to 7 days. He or she then starts use again with a lower dose. If necessary, he or she repeats this process until he or she no longer get the rash. It seems that both of these methods will usually result in a person no longer getting the rash. It does not work for everyone though and so I like the idea of using an over the counter antihistamine, to be done with the problem altogether. Rashes also seem to be, to some extent, dose dependent.

CHAPTER TWENTY

Precautions, Dos and Don'ts

Hydration is very important. No matter what the DNP dose is, a person will be more dehydrated than usual. Of course, the larger the dose, the more dehydrated a person will be and the more important it is to drink water. Most DNP users report drinking 1-3 gallons of water a day.

First time users should always start with lower doses. Everyone is different and it is better to find out how an individual reacts to DNP on lower doses. 200 mgs at most is what is generally recommended for the first three days. After that time, doses can be slowly increased. I personally would hope no one would go over 400mg a day for any reason. I

> "Most DNP users report drinking 1-3 gallons of water a day"

myself used a 200mg a day at first and moved up to 400mg a day. I did go to 600mg a day for the last two days. I took a lot of supplements to counteract the side effects and these were quite effective. Also I used DNP during winter. I was walking around outdoors in 30-degree weather in a tee shirt and feeling comfortably warm. These doses in the summer would be a different experience, I am sure. I would think based on clinical studies, that for almost anyone, 200mg a day would be high enough to achieve excellent results.

DNP and Eating

DNP does not suppress hunger like Ephedrine and many other thermogenics. DNP actually causes an increase in hunger, because it is burning fat. This increase is often described by DNP users as strong carbohydrate cravings.

This problem is often and effectively solved with appetite suppressants. In my opinion it is not even necessary as the fat burning is so great, that even a daily caloric intake, that is a little over maintenance levels, can allow for a tremendous fat loss at 200-400mg a day. DNP will still burn fat as long as a person doesn't pig out and overeat tremendously.

Diuretics

No one should ever take diuretics while on DNP! A strong diuretic, like Lasix, taken while on higher doses of DNP could be disastrous. As I have stated before, I am not a medical doctor and cannot give medical advice, but from my research I believe diuretics and DNP should never be mixed. Any water retained during a DNP cycle clears in less than week. Please be patient.

DNP should not be used by anyone who is going to have to spend extended periods of time in warm conditions, such as someone who has to work outdoors in hot weather. The same is true, if someone is going to be exerting himself strenuously for extended periods of time.

It is important to replenish electrolytes lost through sweating while on DNP. Gatorade® and V8® juice are great sources for potassium. Sodium and Magnesium are both needed as well.

CHAPTER TWENTY-ONE

Modern Use Cycle Logs

This section is comprised of records kept by two modern day DNP users. Their first hand experiences with DNP are kept in the form of a log. Like these men, many modern DNP users are body builders and it is common for them to keep public logs of their cycles of DNP use, and also steroid, growth hormone and other cycles of substances they use.

They keep these public records often on a daily basis in real time throughout their cycle to share information and results for the benefit of other body builders. These logs are often as compelling as they are informative. I have read literally hundreds of logs and found them and the interaction they engender to be often humorous, dramatic and even inspiring.

These particular logs were not kept real time online, so there is none of the normal interaction between these men keeping the logs and the readers. Other than that, they are fairly typical logs. This first log is very close in duration and dosing to my own first time DNP use.

Intro

First things first. This is my take on my DNP. Please don't take it as instructions on what to do or how to do it - its simply my experience of DNP.

Currently will be running 200mg DNP for 3 days and then 400mg

DNP for the next 6. Total of about 9-10 days. Meals mostly consist of oats and whey, fishcakes chicken and veg, chicken and veg, chicken sarnies, loads and loads of water (6-8 litres), few pints of milk and tea & coffee. In between meals, there is fruit.

Day 1- 12th June

Took 200mg just before bed. Taken with water and some adex i'm taking as anti-bloat and anti-gyno for tren/test. Had a Disturbed nights sleep. Lots of tossing and turning and feeling too warm. Not sure if it was all in my head. During the day, felt very thirsty all day. Drank 8-9 500ml bottles of water and half a 2 litre bottle of sprite amongst my normal food. Feeling a little sickly this evening after my work out. TBH the whole work out I felt drained. This is gonna be a hard 10 days. Got some V8 this evening to help top me up. Will be taking a cocktail of vits to keep me full of all of the essentials. TBH, can't seem to drink enough water on this stuff! 17 stone 1lb.

Day 2- 13th June

Took 200mg just before bed. Slept fine. Drunk lots of water today. Same pretty much as yesterday. Feel a little after each meal. Weight has dropped a little to about 16 stone 12/13lbs. Body shape looks somehow different, GF commented on it.

Day 3- 14th June

Took 200mg just before bed. Slept fine. Can't eat or drink enough today. Have drunk about a gallon of water to day including a 2 litre bottle of water in about 2 hours, prolly less. Lips feel dry, really need to drink more. Also need to eat a little more. Now, each time I eat, I get 30-40 mins of feeling warm. Its actually quite nice and very
204

bearable. In fact, I would say i'm not even having to 'bare' it at the mo. Its quite do-able. Weight has bobbed back up to 17 stone on the nose. Slightly bloated look, but still looking more trim than I was. Always hungry, always thirsty. Lips are quite dry if I don't drink up enough.

Day 4- 15th June

Took 200mg just before bed. Slept fine. 200mg taken in the morning. Feeling warm but totally bearable. Will need to wear light fitting clothes this week in the office. Drank about 2 litres this morning in about 1.5 hours. Don't know if it was the DNP but I had some really really mad lucid dreams last night about making it with some posh totty - really strange as i'm really happy with my GF! Think the warmth on day one was all in my head. I feel warm now, but not as hot as I was. Will be taking the little one swimming today. Will be nice and cool! **update** A couple of hours after taking tab i'm properly toasty! Again its actually quite nice, quite bearable. Defo know its there/happening tho! Pool was freezing since i'm nice and warm LOL!

Day 5- 16th June

Took 200mg just before bed. Slept fine. 200mg taken in the morning. Feeling warmer but still totally bearable. Drank about 5 litres today. Ate plenty, feeling warm. Back is sweaty and so is arse. Warm on face and belly. Still get a burn after each tab and after each meal. Seems to be good working all the time. Always hungry. GF has commented that i'm always sounding like i'm breathing heavily which I can say i've also noticed. Losing fat slowly - ex commented how I was looking slimmer when I dropped the baby off yesterday. Had the tab earlier than I had before. Burn feels better, nice and warm! Fat melting away. Starting seeing definition all over, esp on the chest and arms. Gotta admit i'm really enjoying the use of DNP!

Day 6- 17th June

Took 200mg at about 8pm. Slept fine. 200mg taken in the morning. Drank another 4-5 litres during my working day. Breath tastes terrible altho the misses says there is nary a smell to it. To me it feels like i've eaten dog turd which I can assure you isnt nice. Weight 1st thing in morning is 16 stone 10lbs, so i'm down about 4-5lbs since the beginning, which is encouraging. I have bloated in the last day or two but there is more shape to me like I said yesterday but i'm less vascular than I was closer to the beginning of the cycle. Always feeling warm now, but its not at all bad and at no point so far thought 'Wtf am I doing here?'. Keep getting sore joints at the moment, esp my hips 1st thing in the morning and also bizarrely in my left thumb. The GF did wake me last nite because she thought I was breathing heavily, but at all points i've felt fine and altho I currently breathe harder, i'm not feeling like i'm about to pass out or anything. Starting to be able to smell sulphur today. May even had a faint whiff of it yesterday.

Day 7- 18th June

Took 200mg just before bed. Slept fine. 200mg taken in the morning. Did sleep a little more sweaty than normal. Beyond that, fine. Weight now 16 stone 7lbs, when considering water bloat - is fab! Was quite closed today so felt quite clammy for most of the day which wasn't the nicest feeling that i've ever had tbh! Did an arm workout (first whilst on 400mg DNP) this evening. My fcuking god how hard was that!? I sweated thro it, altho looking considerably more vascular and lean then before, it felt like I was lifting twice the weight. I came out the gym, having completed one our absolutely covered, glistening head to food with sweat (look good in the mirrors tho LOL!). I'm now sitting typing this at 11pm absolutely drained, feeling dead on my feet. I could tell the DNP was leaching extra oxygen for the muscle since I was breathing so heavily. When I stopped to hydrate myself every so often I drank at the same time as gulping for much needed oxygen.
206

Feeling a little flat as my muscle is empty (or at least feels it) of any real glycogen stores. Starting to look forward to coming off. Not because of the DNP heat or sweat or the like - I just hate feeling so weak on it!

Day 8- 19th June

Took 200mg just before bed. Slept fine. 200mg taken in the morning. Can smell sulphur all the time now and even taste it. Which is a bit strange but down to the DNP. Also getting lots of hard lumps of snot at the back of my nose. Still, I still haven't any problems dealing with the heat. All is going fine TBH. Enjoying this - at 16 stone 7lbs, the weight loss has been mental and this is whilst holding water as well. The misses commented today that at night I radiate heat and its uncomfortable for me to be close to her. I do sweat at night, but its no worse than tren sweats that i've had before and is more than easy to cope with. Trained well tonite on my shoulders and I actually enjoyed it, weights were almost normal despite carbs being eaten away by the DNP!

Day 9- 20th June

Took 200mg just before bed. Slept fine. 200mg taken in the morning. Sweated, tossed and turned last nite. Felt very hot and uncomfortable unlike before on this cycle of DNP. Made the mistake of eating a load of cookies today (since DNP will burn it off) and fcuk me have I been hot. All day in the office, sweat dribbled down my back, all day my legs have felt slimy, all day has my head itched and my back felt clammy. Hell, even my nose feels itchy FFS! Sitting here typing this topless and legs feeling slimy. Will not make the mistake of eating this many carbs next cycle of this amazing compound. I have decided today to make today my last of DNP. Not because of the heat, but so I can have it out of my system for the start of the next working week -

its been close in the office due to the moisture in the air and i'd rather be working comfortably for the sake of a few hours. I've already lost 7-8lbs before the water weight comes off so i'm happy. End weight before water loss is 16 stone 6/7lbs.

Conclusion

Very good, very manageable compound. Its very easy to work out if you are eating too many carbs (you burn up!) and very quick to see and feel the effects. Its not as lethal as has been made out. In my readings ahead of time, I discovered the lethal dose is stupidly high - something like 333mg/kg of body weight - you'd have to be nuts to consume that amount (altho bear in mind the 48 hour half life does causes it to stack up quickly but it would be very hard in my option to get near that figure (that would be around 16 tabs a day at 200mg/tab on day 1!). Next cycle I may take it higher than 2 tabs at 200mg per tab a day, to 3 tabs at 200mg to see if that fat loss is better, but any more and i'd advise having the time off work, somewhere you can relax and keep cool. At 400mg per day, I found it easy to live with, I actually enjoyed all the water I was drinking (skin loved it) and the weight loss was second to none. I wouldn't recommend it to anyone as simply its a very personal compounds - from the reading i've done, everyone reacts in a different way to it. Me, I react well for fat loss, and well for heat. For some people it just knocks them out of actually being able to live normally. Interestingly mind you, I normally prefer to be cold rather than hot and yet I didn't have problems, which I found unusual but pleasing.

I'd also advise to have a spare set of bed clothes to hand so every couple of days you can change the sheet and wash them. I didn't and the bed stinks of my sweat. I felt fine (yet warm) and realise I sweated a lot (was nasty getting out of bed for a p1ss and coming back in and lying on cold sweat!). Don't expect to be able to train normally - your body is completely drained of carbs (or at least feels it) and very
208

quickly you want to stop (I pushed through it) and feel drained. Lower the weights a little, take your time and drink lots. Even in this time in the gym, i've read you'll be burning around 150% of the normal cals for the exercise. Didn't even try to do any cardio for this cycle. Every day I felt a little breathless and wouldn't want to push it and feel dizzy and maybe even throw up - you dont want to risk your body going warm when your hypothalamus kicks in and tries to help out makes you feel worse!

Pictures will be up as soon as i've completed the cycle and had a few days for the water to drain and the carbs to kick back in - i'm feeling really rather flat right now and very puny.

Any questions, just ask!

All the best,
Papa

Epilogue

TBH I believe the following to be a example and perhaps a good Timetable of Effects and Symptoms of a DNP Cycle, I certainly found it pretty much mirrored my experience:

DNP CYCLE Day 1 -None; possibly elevated carbohydrate cravings and/or temperature elevation.

DNP CYCLE Day 2 - T4-T3 conversion has begun to decrease; lethargy possible. Temperature should be elevated, and radiation of heat is noticeable.

DNP CYCLE Days 3-5 - Body temperature is elevated, with all the effects that one expects from DNP use. In addition, water retention usually becomes manifest here.

DNP CYCLE Days 6-10 - Definite water retention, along with other symptoms of use; user most likely feels fatter due to having "flatter" muscles (mainly the result of glycogen depletion) and holding water. Final DNP dose taken in the evening of Day 10.

DNP CYCLE Days 11-12 - DNP is clearing the system slowly. All symptoms are still present.

DNP CYCLE Days 13-14 - Water should be gone by now, or getting there. Mild diuretics will expedite this. The user will probably notice perceived greater cardiovascular and muscular endurance.

96 Hours After Final Dose - This is when someone tends to look their best. Their glycogen stores are usually compensated at this point and the retained water should be gone.

Second Cycle Log

This man's experience on his DNP cycle is incredibly similar to my own. The only real differences are that he had a little more of a problem with sweating than I did and his cycle was a little more than twice as long. He mistakenly refers to DNP as an anabolic a few times but other than that he was extremely knowledgeable about DNP and the proper protocols to optimally use it. This log is full of valuable information. I think it's rather entertaining too.

You will notice that he was not harmed, thinks it is safe if you don't do something stupid, intends to do it again and doesn't know what all the fuss is about. My sentiments exactly!

Cycle Log:

I'd like to emphasize the fact that I am by no way an expert in this area. I have tried ECA, Clen and T3, as well as SesaPure, Glucorell and Thermorexin (all three together yielded no results at all). The first was the most successful, although still disappointing. Clen gave very little results (even though I was using Spiropent) and I was barely feeling any side effects @ 120mcg per day. I seem to have a very high tolerance to anabolics. This is why I was excited about DNP.

Preparation and planning

My stats at the beginning:

Weight	Height	%Body Fat
103 kg	1m86cm	27
227 lb	6'0"	27

I planned a 25 days cycle. Although I experienced high tolerance to anabolic in the past, I still opted for a slow beginning. First to let my body adapt, second to verify if I had an allergy to DNP. I had some Benadryl here ready to be taken if that was the case. My cycle was planned like this:

Day 1-3: 200mg
Day 4-25: 400mg (in two doses, 1 AM, 1 PM)

The idea behind a lower dose but longer cycle is that the side effects (lethargy for example) are not as present if at all present, and literature suggest it is the most productive way of taking DNP.

What I absolutely did not do during the cycle:
1) Consume any amount of alcohol
2) Stay in hot area for any long period of time

I drank from 4 to 6 liters of water per day, as well a vegetable juice (V8) in the amount of 500ml per day, approx.

I tried to keep an average isocaloric diet, with slightly higher carbs than the rest. I avoided very fat food (like fast food) in my everyday diet, but I did have some nonetheless (twice in fact).

Supplementation

Probably the most important part of all. Before starting I ordered and got everything I needed. The literature defers a lot in that area, so anything that was mentioned at least twice was included in my dietary supplementation.

Morning	Afternoon	Evening
400IU Vitamin E	400IU Vitamin E	400IU Vitamin E
1g Vitamin C	1g Vitamin C	1g Vitamin C
15ml Glycerol	15ml Glycerol	15ml Glycerol
ECA*	ECA*	ECA*
300mg Potassium	300mg Potassium	300mg Potassium
Gluconate	Gluconate	Gluconate

* 200mg Caffeine, 325mg Aspirin, 24mg Ephedrine

Everything was ordered on the net together except the Glycerol, which was obtained in a pharmacy. The Glycerol was a bitch to take…it tastes like grade A shit. I found that 15ml of the stuff, dilated in about 50ml of something very sweet (Coke for example) is the easiest way to take it. Taking it alone or in water means puking. You have been warned.

I was suppose to add Pyruvate here but because USPS messed up and I got it way too late into my cycle and decided to go without it.

Day 1-3

Nothing to say… I took my supplements and just like any other anabolic, I didn't feel a thing with the 200mg of DNP. I had to start taking Benadryl a few days prior to starting the DNP cycle because of summer allergies… so I guess I will never know if I was allergic to DNP.

I've been drinking around 4,5L of water per day, as well as around 1L of Ice Tea, and 500ml of V8. That is around of 6L of liquid alone, and coupled with the Glycerol… well, I literally pee every 15 minutes, and my urine is crystal clear, which means I'm urinating only excess water. I forgot to take my Glycerol on the evening of day 3 and noticed it affected my hydration level a lot: my pee took back its usual pale yellowish color the next morning and I no longer had to go pee every 20 minutes. This shows the importance of the Glycerol, and that in spite of its awful taste, it works well.

Day 4

It was my first day @ 400mg and I was expecting excessive sweating: in vain. There was definitely something happening though. I could feel my body working at a higher pace. My stomach growled all day: I

213

didn't feel at all that hungry. For example, here is what I ate:

Morning:
1x bowl of Special K w/ Dark Chocolate bits cereal. 1x small glass of orange juice

Afternoon:
White rice with chicken in plum sauce with other vegetables. Enough that I was full.

Afternoon snack:
Special K chocolate cereal bar

Evening:
Homemade cheeseburger burger with homemade French fries.

I couldn't tell how much calories this was, but it's about the same intake every day, and I did not specifically increased it for the DNP cycle duration. I suppose ECA helped appetite suppression. In any case, I felt no lethargy. A little bit of sweating perhaps. The weather has been exceptionally cold since I started (18-24 outside) but I have an A/C unit with a fan here once temperatures go up again.

As for my sleep, I have not needed any Melatonin at all, I sleep just fine.

Day 5

I was curious this morning to see if I had lost anything so far. I know the first three days on DNP are slow, while carbs are being depleted and I'm on a relatively low dose anyway. So after I woke up, had my morning visit to the bathroom, I undressed and stepped on the scale: I couldn't believe it.

101.4kg , 25% Bf. That's already almost a 2kg loss and 2% BF loss in 4 days... I still can't believe it, it's actually 1lb/per day as the legend tells, and I haven't felt any of the bad side effects yet. Hopefully I didn't jinx myself and it will stay so effective *knock on wood*.

***

It's now 4 :51PM and OH MY GOD. I ate my lunch at 14h00 today since I woke up early and I started sweating a lot about 45min after I ate. And I had to take a nap because I got so tired ... after the nap I was still sweating but I wasn't tired anymore. I did jinxed myself... whatever

Day 6

I have tried to drink more water today, and it did help. I felt less lethargy, in fact almost none at all, after my lunch. I keep a fan blowing on me while I work to stay comfortable. I keep taking my temperature every 2 hours – but I think my thermometer is of the el-cheapo brand. It says my temp is 36.1C which would suggest hypothermia. I'm definitely not in a hypothermia state!

Something I haven't mentioned yet: DNP cycles will benefit from eating carbs, lots of carbs. They are the activating factor. But the literature suggests you benefit more from simple carbs than complex ones. Hence, during the week, I eat the best simple carb source: fruits. They're healthy and good for the DNP cycle.

During the week-end, I eat candies and chocolate – another source of simple carbs. It feels weird because they hold a lot of calories and seem to go against the purpose of doing a DNP cycle, which is losing weight. But if I don't allow myself to eat some chocolate or sweets, I'm afraid I'll develop a strong craving for it, which wouldn't do me any good. So eating fruits during the week, and candies during the week-end, brings some sort of balance to my appetite and cravings and is fruitful to my DNP cycle.

19h27   —

The lethargy and sweating hit me about 2 hours ago. (Had lunch at 15h30 approx). I napped for an hour and after I woke up I had to put the A/C on, although room temperature is only 24.7C. I just feel warm and not too well.

22h00-

Holy Batman ! The sweating have been constant since my 2nd 200mg dose this afternoon. Since I had been fairly resistant to T3, Clen and ECA, I would have thought the sweating would stay as they were at day 4 and 5, even though the literature said it could take 6-7 days for the sides to really kick in.

Lethargy is no longer present at all. It seems to really hit me for an hour only, about one hour I ingest my 2nd 200mg dose. But I guess the sweating I now feel (I actually don't sweat a lot. In fact, when I was at my most athletic about 3 years ago with 4 Volleyball practices a week and 3 times at the gym, I never sweated a lot. I never even sweat a lot even when my pulse is in the 130 and I'm doing extensive cardio. I'm just really sticky and wet all over my body, but I'm not actually dripping. In fact, it's how I feel after a long cardio session. That tells me DNP is working.) will be like this for the whole cycle. I have turned on the A/C and plan to keep it on at nights. With the A/C on and a fan, I'm comfortable. I even just finished cleaning the whole apartment! As I said, no lethargy.

Also great is that I am able to greatly concentrate to revise for my exams. I was afraid DNP would come in the way. It's not affecting my ability to work or do my usual daily activities. But as I said, A/C is absolutely required.

Finally, I *really* need to eat as soon as I'm a bit hungry, otherwise I start feeling very weak and tired. Nuts, fruits and water are always available to me. I guess with the ECA enhancing the DNP's effects, it is to be expected.

Day 8

Yesterday the sweating started right after the first dose for the first time since I began the cycle, which wasn't that surprising at all. They have not increased and are as described on day 6. The biggest problem is insomnia. I haven't figured yet how to set the A/C all night at a comfortable setting. It's loud and too cold, so I find myself being under the drapes for 1 hour, them I'm too hot and go on top, rinse, repeat. I took one 3mg Melatonin capsule the last two days before bed, and although it helped me to go o sleep the first time, if I wake up during the night (which I did both nights, often) its effects are already gone.

I can only imagine how uncomfortable one must feel on a 600mg dose – my god. I feel quite tired today, but possibly due more to the bad sleep I got (in fact almost none at all) the past two nights than lethargy caused by DNP. During the day while I study or work with A/C and a fan on me there is no real discomfort. I am sticky sure, but it's nothing as bad as some people described (dripping on the floor for example).

I just hope I can find a way to sleep comfortably soon, because I will otherwise not be able to stick to my plan and go another 17 days without sleep. Quite unfortunate, since any other side effects are more than tolerable.

Day 10

Lethargy hasn't been a problem at all since the sweating has been constant from morning to evening. Whether this is because my body adapted or something else I could not say – I haven't changed supplementation at all.

This morning I was alarmed because the scale still showed 101kg/25% bf. However I noticed augmentation in water retention. According to the scale, I've had an increase of 3,5% in water retention, which equals to about 3kg more of additional water being held than normally. This should clear out within 7 days after the cycle ended.

Day 14

I've passed the half cycle mark, and I have not felt any lethargy since day 6. Although I do not officially weight myself except every 5 days (tomorrow will be noted down), I have noted a dramatic increase in fat loss effect for the past 3-4 days. The only possible explanation: T3 has been fully used and depleted in my body. This means enhanced effects, but bad for liver for the next 11 days or so., which is why I would be VERY reluctant to do more than 25 days.

Just for the heck of it I weighted myself after dinner. Since I passed the last 3 days away visiting family, and had forgotten my glycerol, I did not take it for three whole days. Result: scale indicated a 22% BF (5% drop since beginning of cycle) and water level of 58% (a 8% increase than usual, ~50% on normal days). This means I'm holding

218

about 8kg of extra water at the moment. The fact T3 depleted and I missed taking glycerol for three days (a very important component to hydration) possibly explains this drastic change. Since the scale indicated 103KG, and I had just eaten dinner (and was dressed), I estimate the scale tomorrow morning will indicate something around 100KG with a 55% water level (5kg of water), which would mean at day 15 I'd have lost around 8KG in fat (around 17.6lbs), which is close to the ''advertised'' 1lbs-1.5lbs fat loss per day. Not so surprising since I am taking an ECA stack with the DNP.

So is it working? Apparently, it is. Is it worth it? So far I am inclined to say so. I have felt no lethargy at all, but the sweating is constant and immensely annoying. Since you sweat all day (and I am not one to sweat a lot, those who could actually water plants after 45min of cardio will hate DNP for that) it is just very uncomfortable. A/C is for me an absolute necessity: with a fan blowing on my pores I will not be as wet (if at all) but will feel warm nonetheless. As soon as I get outside, or I'm at University studying, you can actually feel the sweat sliding down your back – a very annoying side effect. It is important to mention, although you feel warm, it doesn't actually mean you have fever. I take my temperature every 6 hours and have never been above 37,4C even though I felt I was standing on an erupting volcano. If you do experience fever, you must stop taking DNP immediately until fever is gone.

All side effect(s) aside, needless to say, I'm looking forward end results after this cycle

Day 21

Lack of updates because I was too busy. Because I had started to feel less and less sweating and curious at seeing the effects, I added a

200mg dose in the evening to bring the total dosage to 600mg. I did sweat a lot more during my sleep, but A/C and a fan, I just stayed on top of the covers and it was ok. I noticed I sleep better on my side, because if I lie on my back, I'm guaranteed to wake up in a very wet bed the next morning.

Day 22

Since there is only 3 days left to my cycle I decided to keep up the 600mg and see where it leads me...

Day 23

Ok, no lethargy, more sweating for sure. I have neglected my glycerol a lot in the past 10 days, sometimes forgetting it 2 times out of 3, and I've noticed the DNP to be less effective. I suspect my DNP to be either a little under dosed, or I don't eat enough carbs (I try to eat a lot of fruits for simple carbs).

I'm anxious to see results at the end of the cycle.

Day 25

Yesterday was my last day because I got food poisoning and threw up a few times during the night my dinner. It was actually pasta from a very good restaurant, but I was not aware they were 2 days from closing for 1 month summer vacation: I properly got some old sauce or something. Anyway since I was already pretty dehydrated after the throwing up and weak, I stopped the cycle one day short. Would have been the stupidest thing ever to take DNP after being sick. I pondered about the idea of maybe if it was the DNP that made me sick, but my symptoms were really of food poisoning. I re-hydrated myself slowly, re-balanced electrolytes and one day later I was back to normal.

I will wait around a week before releasing the journal, I need to give my body time to stabilize and water retention to become normal again.

5 days post-cycle

My stats post-cycle:

Weight	Height	%Body Fat
94.4kg	1m86cm	23
208lbs	6'0"	23

My BF has settled at 23% and my weight at around 95KG. I am a bit disappointed, but not entirely. I mean towards the end I didn't watch what I ate carefully, I pretty mucha te anything I wanted and try to eat as much simple carbs from fruits as possible.

I've lost 8KG which is around 18lbs in 24 days, which turns out to be around 0.75lbs of fat loss per day. My BF is still high though, I'm surprised I didn't lose more than that, but again – my scale was only 100EUR so it's not actually the most accurate tool.

Conclusion

Can I say my DNP cycle was worth it ? Absolutely. 18 pounds in 24 days is still impressive (even if not on part with the 1lb/day legend).

A resume of my side effects:
- Sweating
- Partial Insomnia

That's it. I want to say something about insomnia. I did sleep, but never very deep and well. This past week I have had marvelous nights of sleep, in fact one night I was so deep asleep that the three alarms I had set never woke me, as well as my friend who called me on my phone, and as well as the mailman who rang at my door to try and deliver a package. Usually the buzzer makes me jump because it's so loud... I was never that hard asleep in my entire life. If you are familiar with sleep cycles, there is a light, medium and deep level for every cycle, and each cycle renders particular brain functions. The deepest level is what allows maximum resting and is when we dream the most. During the night you go through a few of those cycles. I believe the DNP kept me from ever reaching the deep level of all my sleep cycles (if not all many) because of the sweating and the high metabolic activity (reaching the deepest level requires a particular heartbeat and metabolic speed). It really showed post cycle ....

I felt no lethargy except the first days. Sweating was by far the most annoying factor. I am not one to sweat a lot, and since it was revision time, I was almost at home in the A/C in a cold room, so I didn't sweat. But as soon as I got out, it would start. Nights were also annoying since you can never sleep fully well, but I never felt exhausted nor tired, just not over the top relaxed like when you had one of those amazing night sleep.

People are afraid of DNP because they don't understand. There is no physical possibility for DNP to kill you by its mechanism alone, rather the side effect it creates which is severe dehydration because of it intervenes directly within the mitochondria's Krebs cycle of ATP production (google NA/k ATPase or Krebs cycle to understand more how it works) rather than through hormonal messages like ECA or Clen works. Therefore, if you're not an idiot and are aware of the extreme importance of hydrating (through liquid glycerol or glycerol effervescent tablets (used in patients recuperating from severe dehydration after severe diarrhea for example)) and avoid diuretics there is no real danger.

The only real danger is idiocy or a severe overdose. Both factors are dangerous for many other anabolic or drug. I have to say after having using it; I don't understand the paranoia behind it.

Finally because I do yearly clinical immersion for weeks, I had a blood test made post cycle, and everything looked OK.

My next cycle

Because of T3 depletion, the liver has it at its hardest. I am no expert in anabolics or steroids but since I am a medical student I do know how the naturally produced hormones affect the body. Although T3 suppression for a short while (in my case around 12 days) will not kill the thyroid gland nor put me in a state of hypothyroidism, the fact the body doesn't have T4 or T3 for a while (T3 is the physiology active hormone) affects some organs (nothing extreme). I will leave at least 30 days before my next cycle, and after 10 days my thyroid functions should have returned to normal.

Meanwhile I need to analyze what I did wrong and try to be more efficient... perhaps a 14 days cycle this time, with day 1-2 on 400mg, then days 3-14 on 600mg. Since I didn't sweat more with 400 vs 600 (I just sweat longer during the night) I could minimize the annoyance of having 24 days of sweating and supplement taking. Besides, it's easier to stay on the carb plan and remain disciplined for 14 days then 24 days!

CHAPTER TWENTY-TWO

Final Word

This book has kept its promise. I have proven that DNP is the most effective fat reduction therapy known. I have proven that DNP does no harm to the body. Along with these two truths, I have also proven through logic and clinical reports, that there is no reason to keep this substance from the American people.

I have also shown the reality, that sadly, greed and self-interest are the only things that stand between the American public and this amazing weight-loss substance.

For the purpose of adequately assessing the terrible price the American public is paying for this tragic injustice, let's imagine what would happen if DNP were returned to legal status as a prescription medicine. Overweight people could take a pill and comfortably and safely lose weight in basically the same way they would with aerobic exercise at the rate of around 10 pounds a month. In a few years, there would be almost no overweight people left. America would be healthier, happier more beautiful; A dream come true for countless millions, but a financial nightmare for the weight-loss and medical industries.

Who is winning this contest of interests and the sad role manipulation of governmental power plays in this tragedy, have been brought to light. Will this knowledge of these truths lead to the just victory of the American People being given this providentially perfect fat reduction therapy? Or will the few intrepid Americans, successfully using DNP, in spite of FDA fiat and caprice, continue to be forced to be **Illegally Thin**?

Where to Obtain DNP:

These guys are US based. They sell DNP at a very good price as a bulk powder. If you order from them they will require a copy of your driver's license and a letter explaining what you want to use it for. As far as I know DNP is not a scheduled substance. I wonder what the government's interest is in intimidating people from buying a substance that is not scheduled?

Sciencelab.com

Here is the URL to the order page

http://www.sciencelab.com/page/S/PVAR/10411/SLD3364?gclid=C KOEgteonZECFQmgGgodoGsaPg

These guys manufacture DNP and a handful of related substances as dyes. I would assume it could be purchased at little more than the cost of dirt at higher volumes from them.

Henan Luoran Co.,Ltd.

Add:	Guxian Town, Yanshi,luoyang City ,Henan Province
Contact:	Zhangwei

Tel:	+86-379-65226166
Fax:	+86-379-65226169
Web Site:	http://www.luoran.com

There are many suppliers around the world that sell DNP in capsule form. I have not given any of the supplier's names because I cannot attest to their reliability. These companies I have given are selling for commercial/industrial uses and though I have never received any DNP from either they seem reliable enough.

References

1. Horner, Warren D. "A Study of Dinitrophenol and its Relation to Formation of Cataract." San Francisco: *Arch Ophthal.* 1942 Jun. Vol 27(6):1097-1121.1942

2. Tainter, Maurice L. Cutting, Windsor C. and Stockton B. "Use off Dinitrohenol in Nutritional Disorders, A Critical Survey of Clinical Results" *American Journal of Public Health Nations Health.* 1934 Oct. Vol 24(10): 1045-53.

3. Bell, Jacques. "Biological Study of Dinitro Drugs in Humans." *Etude biologique des produits dinitres chez l'homme. Medecine.* 1939. 19:749-54. Translation © 1996 Robert Ames

4. United States Patent *4,673,691* Bachynsky June 16, 1987 This whole study can be analyzed in more detail in the clinical studies section of this book.

5. Bagchi, Debases and Preuss, Harry G. Obesity: *Epidemiology, Pathophysiology, and Prevention.* CRC Press. 2007.

6. "2,4-Dinitrophenol." http://en.wikipedia.org/wiki/2,4-Dinitrophenol

7. "2,4-Dinitrophenol." http://mesomorphosis.com/steroid-profiles/dnp.htm

8. Koizumi M, Yamamoto Y, Ito Y. Takano M, Enami T, Kamata E. Hasegawa R. "Comparative study of toxicity of 4-nitrophenol and 2,4-dinitrophenol in newborn and young rats." *Journal of Toxicological Sciences.* 2001. Vol 26 (5). 299-311.

9. Looney J.M. and Hoskins R.G. "The Therapeutic Use of Dinitrophenol and 3:5 Dinitro-Ortho-Cresol in Schizophrenia." *American Journal of Psychiatry.* 1935 Mar. Vol 91. 1009-1017. ©1935 American Psychiatric Association.

10. Ru K, Taub ML, Wang JH. "Specific inhibition of breast cancer cells by antisense poly-DNP- oligoribonucleotides and targeted apoptosis." *Oncology Research.* 1998. Vol 10(8). 389-397.

11. Gabai VL. "Inhibition of uncoupled respiration in tumor cells. A possible role of mitochondrial Ca2+ efflux." *FEBS Lett.* 1993 Aug. Vol 329(1-2). 67-71.

12. Bystryn JC, Perlstein J. "Autocatabolism of surface macromolecules shed by human melanoma cells." *Cancer Res* 1982 Jun; 42(6):2232-7.

13. Burd R, Wachsberger PR, Biaglow JE, Wahl, ML, Lee I, Leeper DB. "Absence of Crabtree effect in human melanoma cells adapted to growth at low pH: reversal by respiratory inhibitors." *Cancer Res.* 2001 Jul. Vol 61(14). 5630-5.

14. Sedan, Jean. "A propos de deux cas de cataracte par phenols dinitres." *Annales d'Oculistes.* (Concerning Two Cases of Cataract Caused by

Dinitrophenol)1939. 176-191. Translation Copyright 1996 by Robert Ames.

15. "Lipitor."http://www.lipitor.com/about-lipitor/side-effects.jsp?source=google&HBX_PK=s_lipitor+side+effects&HBX_OU=50&o=23127370|166376222|0

16. http://www.drugs.com/pro/hydrocodone-and-acetaminophen-elixir.html

17. "Adderall." http://www.drugs.com/adderall.html

18. *United States v. Sean Zhang* (E.D.N.Y.) June 25, 2002.

19. "2,4-Dinitrophenol." http://www.scorecard.org/chemical-profiles/html/24dinitrophenol.html

20. Hecht, Annabel and Janssen, Wallace. "Diet Drug Danger Déja Vu." *FDA Consumer*. 1987 Feb. Republished on quackwatch.com on Jan 29, 2003.

21. "FDA and Pharma's Death Toll-Reform or Business as Usual?" 14 June 2007. Sept 2008. http://www.newmediaexplorer.org/sepp/2007/06/14/fda_and_pharmas_death_toll_reform_or_business_as_usual.htm.

22. Lawson, Gary W. "Impact of User Fees (i.e. Drug Industry Money) on Changes within the FDA." Public Administration Doctoral Thesis. May 2005. Sept 2008. http://www.fdastudy.com/Thesis.htm.

23. Hudgins, Edward L. "Kessler's FDA: An Autopsy."

24. Faloon, William. "FDA Suffers Second Massive Legal Defeat in 'Pearson vs. Shalala II.' Court to FDA, The First Amendment Must Be Followed." LE Magazine. May 2001. Sept 2008. http://www.lef.org/magazine/mag2001/may2001_cover_pearson2_1.html.

25. Health Freedom Protection Act. (H.R. 2117). May 2, 2007. Full text available at http://www.govtrack.us/congress/billtext.xpd?bill=h110-2117.

26. Fox, Stephen. "Resolving The Worsening Crisis At the United States Food and Drug Administration." 15 June 2007. Sept 2008.http://apostille.us/news/resolving_the_worsening_crisis_at_the_united_states_food_and_drug_administration.shtml

27. Kay, Joseph. "The Vioxx scandal: damning Senate testimony reveals drug company, government complicity." 22 Nov 2004. Sept 2008. http://www.wsws.org/articles/2004/nov2004/viox-n22.shtml.

About the Author

Random Knight is a pen name. The author has elected to give his family the protection of anonymity from the millions of people who will feel financially threatened by the truths revealed in this book. He does stand behind every word in this book. He is willing to meet any expert(s) in any appropriate forum to discuss, defend or debate the positions he takes and the truths he reveals in this book. He can be contacted at knightworks@live.com.

Copies of this book and more information on the subject matter included can be found at www.illegallythin.com